Blaze

Advance Praises

The never-say-die attitude of Divyansh should be an inspiration for young and old people from all walks of life. The body may be diseased but, in John Milton's words, 'the mind is its own place and in itself, can make a heaven of hell, a hell of heaven.' Despite his critical illness, Divyansh was able to achieve so much. Truly inspiring and moving. May he continue to find peace wherever he is now.

Sachin Tendulkar,
Bharat Ratna and Former Indian Cricketer

This is a tragic story of a young boy who fought cancer and lost. This is also a sad book, written by the mother of that young man, who did her best by him, only to realize that it was not enough. Not enough to save him. And yet, reading the book right in the midst of the deadliest pandemic the world has perhaps seen, I felt hope. I felt hope, courage and faith—the three things that can survive the greatest tragedies that life (and destiny) can send our way. I saw, even if it was for a fleeting moment, the incredible might of the creative moment. That incredible heart-stopping moment we all—poets, philosophers, painters, storytellers, dreamers—live for. When we try to stare down death and seek immortality through our words, images, dreams, hopes.

Young Divyansh did exactly that. And that is how I discovered his brave story: through his writings, the words he crafted with such infinite care so that the world would remember his life not because he passed away so young, with so much talent, so much love in his heart, but in the hope that however brief our lives are, we can make every moment incandescent with faith.

I will not quote him here. His words will live on through this wonderful book that his mother has written with the support of his father. There are enough quotes in the book to last you an entire lifetime. Cancer can kill a 22-year-old boy but it can never conquer his spirit to live and that is exactly what this book extols. Divyansh has touched immortality with his words.

And that is why I loved reading his story. The story of a young boy I have never met, never seen, never heard of. Yet he could have been my son, my younger brother, my friend. He could have been any one of those bright-eyed, fresh-faced young people who cross your path in the street every day. Nidhi and Sushil have made his story so touching, so incredibly endearing that when you finish reading this book, you will also (like me) feel bereaved.

Today, as I write these words, I grieve for a young man I never knew but who touched my life and passed by into eternity. I grieve for his parents. But at the same time, I feel the incredible power of a life so well lived amidst every adversity. I celebrate the chronicle of his life, his words, the love he shared with everyone during his brief eventful sojourn on this earth.

May his life, his words be an inspiration for all of us who are missing our loved ones in the midst of this pandemic. Let this book be read by every parent who grieves the loss of a son or daughter so that they may have the courage and the grit to face life thereafter. Not with sadness but with a sense of wonderment.

Padmashri Pritish Nandy,
Poet, Journalist and Eminent Media Personality

As I turned the last page over, I was left with the resonance of just how incredible the human spirit is, how vulnerable yet how strong and resilient love can make us, how much courage one can muster for a fight that matters, how much one is willing to sacrifice to gain something more precious than all the riches in the world: that is, time with the person we love.

Farhan Akhtar,
Film Actor

Blaze is the story of young man, Divyansh Atman, and his courageous battle with leukaemia. He was an individual extraordinarily mature beyond his physical age and had the sensitivity of a poet. Apart from the unfairness of it all, I was struck by the positivity with which Divyansh and his mother and the whole family dealt with his illness. Divyansh wrote, 'You see, adversity is a poison with its own antidote.'

The bond between Divyansh and his mother, and between him and his whole family is truly precious and he has put his emotion about it in many poems.

The title of the book has been taken from a poem written by Divyansh with the same name. That poem talks about the unquenchable divine fire present in every person's soul—the fire that grows so bright and radiant resides inside all of us: 'Look into the fire my friends and rekindle the fire in you.'

A cancer specialist runs the risk of becoming immune to the suffering of patients, possibly as a self-protective reflex. However, I must confess that towards the end of the book, I was in tears, with a lump in my throat. Reading *Blaze* has been a spiritually uplifting experience for me. I am happy that his mother is publishing this book so that many more can read it and learn about the enlightened soul that was Divyansh.

Professor Shailesh V. Shrikhande,
Deputy Director, Tata Memorial Hospital;
Head of Cancer Surgery,
Tata Memorial Centre, Mumbai

Divyansh's journey is one of strength, courage and discovery. He was a brave young man who dealt with adversities with faith and hope and shared his talent and deep thoughts through heartfelt poems. The impact of his sincere work and loving words remain long after the reader has finished reading the book.

Padmashri Sudha Murty,
Chairperson, Infosys Foundation

Divyansh Atman's story gives a new beacon of light to the people who are suffering from negative thoughts and proves to be an incredible example of positivity and hope. As Gautam Buddha has said, 'The mind is everything. What you think, you become.' Divyansh proved to the world that no matter the circumstances, talent and creativity know no bounds. When I heard Divyansh's story, I was moved beyond words. Reading his poetry, I was astonished by the raw talent and energy that he carried in his verses. As an artist, I am inspired by Divyansh's story and I hope it can be a source of motivation to everyone who is suffering from a difficult time in their lives. He may not be here with us today but his pure smile and the legacy he has left behind for all of us through his kind words will continue to inspire us eternally.

Padmashri Paresh Maity,
Painter

Thank you for giving the world this gift. This is story of an immortal life.

Divyansh invigorates us every day, inspiring us to be happy and live to our fullest beyond the physical forms.

Vikas Khanna,
Indian Chef and Philanthropist

Blaze is the heartfelt story about a divine soul. It's a narrative of love generously peppered with fortitude. It is a tribute and testament to light in darkness and strength in suffering. As I sadly limped through the pain of Divyansh and his parents, the strong resolve of his spirit extended an insight into my own journey. The courage, love, maturity and insight Divyansh displayed through his heart-breaking journey shows that heartbreak can be accompanied with peace and sorrow with fortitude. There is always a breathtaking pride one feels when one manages to glimpse a never-say-die spirit. And it is one among the myriad emotions that truly stood out for me. Divyansh had a way with words that truly brought out his boundless strength. Some of the lines that he has written remain etched in my mind:

Adversity is
A poison with its own antidote.

And the two lines that tear apart man-made barriers to show our common humanity:

'Are you a Hindu or Muslim?'
'I am hungry...'

These are thoughts that will stay with me.
Blaze is a must read for all.

Dr Yusuf Merchant,
Head of DAIRRC (NGO) and Author of *Happyness*

Blaze is a moving and inspiring story, told with unflinching honesty. Divyansh Atman's zest for life shines through in this book. Nothing, not even a life-threatening illness, could stop him from offering strength to loved ones or trying to achieve his dreams of studying abroad and becoming an engineer. Divyansh's deeply philosophical approach to his illness found expression in the memorable poems he wrote; he presented one of these with confidence at the 100 Thousand Poets for Change festival in Mumbai. Through his words, deeds, will power and optimism, Divyansh kept himself going during the most trying times and profoundly impacted the lives of the people around him. Divyansh's life was snatched away too soon, but as he faced his illness with rare courage and determination, he left behind an important message—that negativity is the true cancer. His positive approach in the face of terrible adversity is a lesson for us all.

Menka Shivdasani,
Poet and Coordinator, 100 Thousand Poets for Change, Mumbai

I feel small after reading the facts about the prodigy Divyansh Atman, who departed at only 22. Perhaps the Lord needed him more.

Shirsendu Mukhopadhyay, Decorated Bengali Author

When life comes close to death, it blossoms like a flower with many petals. There is a Tibetan Buddhist concept: 'Learn death if you want to live a perfect full life'. This is like two poles meeting.

I remember a couple of lines from Emily Dickinson:

A wounded deer leaps highest,
I've heard the hunter tell,
'Tis but the ecstasy of death,
And the brake is still.

Death, not God, is the creator. Every moment extinguished a lamp to light another anew. Death is the nest. Life is a bird. Sky is the limit.

'Divya' means pure, divine. 'Ansha' is a part. When combined, it produces a message: We are the flower, thou the Sun.

Sanjib Chatterjee,
Noted Bengali Author

Blaze
A Son's Trial By Fire
A True Story

Nidhi Poddar
and Sushil Poddar

RUPA

Published by
Rupa Publications India Pvt. Ltd 2021
7/16, Ansari Road, Daryaganj
New Delhi 110002

Sales centres:
Allahabad Bengaluru Chennai
Hyderabad Jaipur Kathmandu
Kolkata Mumbai

ISBN: 978-93-91256-81-4

First impression 2021

10 9 8 7 6 5 4 3 2 1

The moral right of the authors has been asserted.

This book would not have been possible without Divyansh Atman, who gave us the reason to write.

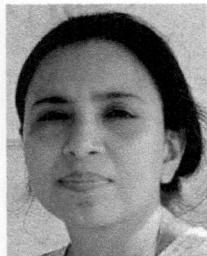

NIDHI PODDAR is a woman of intrepid character who had to pass through ceaseless formidable challenges in her life while parenting her stout and inspiring son, Divyansh Atman, the protagonist of the story. These challenges eventually transformed a homemaker into an author of this book. Nidhi graduated in Economics from Patna University in 1994. She is married to Sushil Poddar and they have a daughter.

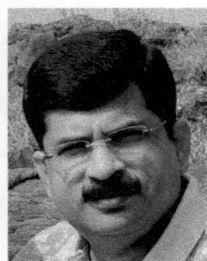

SUSHIL PODDAR is a senior government officer who has been serving his department for the last 27 years. He did his B.Tech from ISM (IIT), Dhanbad in 1989. After serving the mining industry for five years, he joined the civil services in 1994.

Can a disease, more importantly, cancer, be a potent tool of self-evolution for both, the person who suffers from it, and his/her caregivers, especially parents?

The value of good health is realized when it no more remains with us. The journey to salvage a lost friend can still offer myriad opportunities of redemption and self-discovery. It is up to us how we decide to tread this formidable path leading to self-actualization.

Time has made us realize that it is not fair to stereotype a person suffering from cancer from the point of view of cure or recovery. Many a time, such stereotyping comes from our own society, and sometimes, ironically, from the medical fraternity, for its inability to go beyond a point after which you feel you are condemned and vegetative. All these negativities passively entrap the patients and their loved ones in the viciousness of the disease where they die many times before the actual death. This is the worst form of cancer which has plagued our mindset.

In the case of Divyansh Atman, it was not so. Divyansh was the embodiment of courage and self-determination in the face of adversities. His life journey shows us how the path of opportunities can still be paved in the middle of adversities. He lived a big and meaningful life that made a huge impact on the lives of people around him.

Blaze is an attempt to delineate Divyansh's inspirational life journey and ever-evolving motherhood of his mother alongside. Apt to quote few lines from his poem 'Rebirth':

As I stand at the precipice of this path,
I truly understand,

The true nature of transience,
as it always will be.

CONTENTS

FOREWORD

Amitabh Bachchan
'Pratiksha', 10th North-South Road, Juhu-Parle Scheme, Bombay 400 049.

Blaze: A Son's Trial by Fire

Death is supposedly an act of God. To endure the death of a loved one calls for stretching human endurance beyond limits and delving deep into unimagined reserves of courage. The death of a child for a parent, is indescribable in its pain. Whilst I have been part of scenes on screen where a parent faces the death of a child, even whilst one is aware that that is a make-believe story, art is an imitation of life, and the emotional quotient it extracts from an actor is deep. I cannot even begin to imagine what it must feel like in real life.

Blaze is a story that comes from extreme courage. It tells the tale of young Divyansh Atman, who in the face of death, came through like a seasoned warrior. His spiritual maturity far exceeded his physical age. It is a powerful narrative because it is the voice of his parents, (Nidhi and Sushil Poddar) and especially the mother, that tells this story; they who bore him, and bore his suffering in illness, in equal measure. Without leaning into self-pity, the predominant tone is an assimilation of their darkest hours that they have crystallized through this story into an inspirational journey for the readers. This is an emotional read, but one shall emerge transformed by the triumph of the human spirit.

I commend Nidhi and Sushil Poddar for this display of strength in sharing the story of their son Divyansh Atman with the world. I wish them all the very best in the times to come, and pray they continue to inspire people with the progress of the book.

Amitabh Bachchan

Place : Mumbai
Date : November, 19th, 2020

PREFACE
Khalid Mohamed

There wasn't a moment to lose,
no deferred questions, no belated revelations,
just those experienced in time.
Wisdom couldn't wait for gray hair.
It had to see clearly before it saw the light
and to hear every voice before it sounded.

—Excerpt from 'Our Ancestors' Short Lives'
by Nobel laureate Wisława Szymborska

Divyansh Atman has been an invisible force, an exemplar in my life, and in every life he touched before he entered another realm at the age of 22. For 10 years, he didn't battle with leukaemia— he embraced it, expressing his innermost thoughts and that rare spirit of triumph in poems, short stories, letters and musings.

He could have been an engineer, a poet, a novelist. Clearly a prodigious talent, he has left us a legacy not only of his tender and wise words, but also a story which can inspire those who have experienced loss and tragedy in their myriad forms. And who amongst us hasn't?

I learnt of Divyansh, affectionately called Manu, from his father Sushil Poddar, a man of a few words, in sharp contrast to his son. The father is reserved, resilient and, by his innate personality, I could sense that he doesn't want to disclose his seesawing emotional graph in public. Divyansh's mother, Nidhi, is perhaps the opposite: every particle of her emotions is etched on her face. On meeting them together for the first time, I felt intrusive. No questions could be asked, no gratuitous advice extended, no tokenist so-sorry-to-know tendered.

To see Divyansh, who was then in an unconscious condition at Bombay Hospital, was my intuitive response. I foolishly suggested to Sushil that after seeing his son, we could chat in a hotel bar just facing the hospital. We fixed the time. As soon as I reached home, though, there a realization. I had blundered to the point of inadvertently exacerbating Nidhi's feelings. Could she even allow Sushil and me to down an evening beer while their son was in hospital across the road? When I called up to cancel the appointment, Sushil said gently, 'Thank you. I couldn't say no to you. Nidhi wouldn't have said anything but...' The incomplete sentence was spot-on.

On reading the works of Diyvansh, who would be in and out of hospital medical procedures and yet sit for his examinations at St. Mary's School, there was no question in my heart or mind that they must be published. His writings were lined with clarity. And even between the lines, elements, however faint, of neither self-pity nor physical sufferance could be detected.

Divyansh was discharged from hospital; a little nursing home was set up in his room. Cowardly enough, I didn't have the guts to ask for permission to see him. His younger sister, Ananya, was sitting at the dining table, doing her homework. Here was a perfect family that had been torn asunder, I thought.

I was wrong, because Divyansh in his own style—the Urdu word for it would be 'ada'—was ensuring that there wouldn't be the slightest vestige of a smudge ever on their family portrait. It would shine on forever. He would never leave them bereft; his hand would always go up, 'Present, Sir!'

Moved to the core, I came up with the idea (again a foolish one, in retrospect) of writing a script based on three of Divyansh's stories: one dealing with his conversation with a taxi driver en route to collecting his medical reports from a hospital; the second, a bond between a parrot and the pet dog of his ancestral home in Patna and the third sourced from a note written to his sister Ananya. The interlinked short stories could be a salute to Divyansh and, on a broader scale, to all those children and parents who have contended with such a situation—I say 'situation' in order to not compartmentalize such an occurrence. We could upload the result on YouTube; we could get a streaming channel interested. Sushil responded positively, as it is in his nature to agree rather than be discouraging.

Within a week I completed the three scripts and mailed them to him; he saw some potential in them. On re-reading them, though, I could detect that they were inadequate and did little or no justice to the unspoken heroism of Divyansh, still at home, occasionally showing signs of improvement.

It required no Herculean rethinking on my part to understand that no one could relate Divyansh's unwavering joie de vivre, the depth of his intellect and his unbridled sense of humour as accurately as his parents could. We left it at that. Months elapsed; over the phone, Sushil would say that his son was okay, which was his euphemism for 'Let's hope for the best.' The best, of course, is not enough. Diyvansh left.

Months winged by; the world was locked down following the outbreak of the COVID-19 pandemic. We were in the grip of fear and dread, locked at home, dealing with our isolation in our individual ways. Then, in mid-October, Sushil messaged, 'Can we meet at your convenience?' To be absolutely honest, I seized that moment primarily to get a break, a walk in the garden of the housing colony where the Poddars reside. It is not crowded; the greenery and the oceanfront's evening breeze are refreshing. I couldn't wait to see Sushil on a Sunday evening.

Wearing his benign smile, he was carrying a spiral-bound

book in a cloth bag. In three months, Nidhi and Sushil had personally authored *Blaze: A Son's Trial by Fire*. It was almost as if possessed with divinity, they had written a book, a soul-stirring account of Divyansh's journey from Mumbai to Israel and USA for treatment and, simultaneously, to explore the future prospects of joining an American university for higher studies. 'Here We Go Again' goes the title of one of the chapters, obviously alluding to Divyansh's refrain, as he, accompanied by his parents, travelled meeting doctors and medical experts for lines of treatment and possible cure.

Were they fighting a losing battle? No. Rather, the arduous journeys, one unfortunate incident of misdiagnosis in USA and the generous quality of the doctors, nurses and their own relatives indicate the triumph of Divyansh's will and, as importantly, his mother's combat with inevitable disappointments. Our Divyansh's belief in karma and his proximity to yoga, literature, music and the art of cuisine blossomed fulsomely, as his writing became more artful and stoic.

For the parents, could the profoundly touching book have worked as a catharsis? Before hazarding an answer, let me say that the term 'catharsis' has found a place in everyday language to describe moments of insight or the experience of finding closure. Catharsis is used in the frame of Freudian psychoanalysis. But is it that simple to find closure? Instead, I would like to believe Nidhi and Sushil have found a new beginning to love and to cherish their son anew, a son who can clearly see the light and hear every voice before it sounded.

That conclusion, I have reached from my very own personal experience. I lost my mother, Zubeida, at the age of two. I transcribed her unseen memory into a film screenplay directed by the eminent Shyam Benegal. And the question I continue to be asked is, 'That script must have been a catharsis, you must have found closure.'

On the contrary, my mother, who was 19 years old when she perished in an air crash, was born again for me, within me, with the film *Zubeida*.

We are all made of disparate minds and temperaments. The Poddars could have an entirely different take than mine. Still, from what I have known of them and after reading the book, my heart tells me Divyansh has been born again with *Blaze*.

He may not be there in a corporeal form. He will always be there in his writings and in the memory of his smiles and laughter, against all odds. After all, the sun sets to rise every day and always will.

1

THE ECSTASY

I had been waiting for a long time for this day. Since morning, I had been engrossed in arranging everything meticulously for the house-warming puja. The new house, which I dreamt of making a heavenly abode, had been renovated right under my guidance. During the renovation of the new house, Sushil often had to go to Jerusalem with Divyansh for his follow-up treatment. All my life, I never knew how to venture into designing the interior of a house as I came from a humble middle-class family, where the idea of a house with even a modest interior was considered a luxury. My son Divyansh (his pet name was Manu) had to go through ceaseless life-threatening medical problems when we were living in our old house. I often used to coax Sushil to change our residence as it seemed the Vastu of this house was unfavourable to Divyansh's fortunes. There was a crematorium visible from our living room balcony, the sight of which always stirred in me a strange feeling: that whatever misfortunes he was facing, it could be because of this too. Finally, we got another government accommodation, which was bigger and better located. And with this, I thought the fate of my son would change its course for the better. I grabbed the opportunity to explore all my creative senses and put them into the making of the warmest abode for my children. I wanted to infuse my motherly affection and devotion into each and every brick of the house, enough to ward bad spells off my children. The house was ready; we were all set to move homes in December 2016.

After the puja, the priest told us the Vastu of the house was spot-on and prophesied that it would turn the tide in our favour. Divyansh was looking better then. His energy levels were much improved. He would take keen interest in household matters and would often indulge in doing essential shopping to lighten the burden of his father. He devoted a lot of time to Ananya to help her with her studies and take her out for recreational activities. He religiously made it a point to participate in the morning and evening tea sessions with us, adding a sublime shade to our togetherness. He resumed attending his engineering college. I gradually started shedding the bitter memories of the past. I started looking at myself again in the mirror and made attempts to look better in this new lease of life. Whenever Divyansh left for college, I would go right up to the elevator to proudly bid him goodbye. Actually, that was more than just a goodbye. It was my way of fortifying him with my blessings and lacing him with my love so that when he went out, he could face the world with formidable fortitude. Divyansh was now a fledgling again, acquiring new wings thick and fast to live his life as he may have wanted and to face the world with renewed optimism.

Anshoo's wedding was round the corner. Divyansh, amongst all his cousins, was very close to Anshoo and Mridul for the simple reason that they were the ones who spent the maximum time with him. When I was married, Mridul and Anshoo, who are the sons of Sushil's eldest brother Shankar (I call him Bhaiya), were kids. They were adorable. While we were in Kolkata, they used to come to stay with us often, and I would care for them as I would for Divyansh and Ananya. I saw them growing, shaping their careers and getting married. Mridul got married first. Now, it was Anshoo's turn. Divyansh was in absolute ecstasy at the very idea of participating in his wedding, from his grandparents' home in Patna.

For the past five years, I couldn't take Divyansh to our native place as he was struggling with his medical problems and was going through strict treatment protocol. There was also the possibility of catching infection there, as Sushil always reminded me. To me, like for any mother, Divyansh was my world. Honestly, one of the prime reasons was that I didn't want to expose him to any evil eye there. He had suffered a lot by then. It may seem like a ridiculous thought, but it was as if I were keeping him inside my womb and waiting for the right moment to re-birth him. There was one more reason, I must confess now. Over the course of the treatment process, Divyansh had become overweight because of the side effects of the medicines he was taking. The immediate aftermath of these life-saving drugs was the complete eclipse of his physical beauty. His new appearance reached and struck me through the eyes of others. I used to observe visitors looking at him with sympathetic eyes. Those eyes used to pierce me like a needle would impale skin. Some were so curious, they would ask why he had become like this. That's why I always wished to keep him in my lap, saving him from the inquisitive eyes of visitors. Although he himself was quite nonchalant about it and had transcended himself beyond embarrassment, I used to feel a sense of deprivation at this loss of his boyish beauty. Somewhere deep in my heart, I had taken a vow to take him to Patna only when he regained his lost physical aura. I was craving for it, dying to get it back. Now, five years later, when Divyansh had got his lost, well-toned physique back with a much-matured face, eyes evoking wisdom and a radiant smile, I decided he must now, after so many years, go to Patna with elan. My in-laws, as they were in the twilight of their lives, would always insist on me bringing Divyansh to Patna, a request I couldn't fulfil, for which, I still harbour an impalpable guilt in my heart. I must also admit that because of his medical problems and my capricious thinking, I couldn't allow Divyansh to participate in the weddings of Mridul and his two female cousins earlier. Though Divyansh seemingly nourished a desire to visit his grandparents' home and also to attend his cousins' weddings, he always respected my implicit dilemma and never insisted on it.

Anshoo's wedding gave me an opportunity to redeem myself and get over the guilt I was harbouring. The rejuvenated Divyansh was now all set to touch the land where he was born, where both his paternal and maternal grandparents lived, and where he would meet a band of cousins in the big joint family of his dada and dadi. I was ready to cut the umbilical cord I had tied him with to me so far.

Anshoo's wedding had to be close to my heart. To me, he was just like Divyansh. Over the course of Divyansh's treatment process in the past eight years, I had gradually lost hope on all counts, though Sushil always counselled me that everything would become alright one day. The extent of pessimism in me was so great that I had even stopped dreaming of the day when I would see Divyansh as a groom. With the prospect of Divyansh now participating in this wedding, I wanted to celebrate Anshoo's wedding as I would have done Divyansh's. His wedding was fixed for 22 April 2017. In early January, Anshoo, along with his fiancée Shweta, came to meet us. That time, Mridul also joined us with his wife Mahima. We took Anshoo to a nearby fashion store to select a sherwani for him to wear on his wedding day. As he took the final trial of a light pink sherwani, he looked regal. Perhaps I subconsciously saw a glimpse of Divyansh in him then.

That was the last time that Divyansh, Mridul, Mahima, Anshoo and Shweta were together. That was also perhaps the last time they together resonated blissfulness. And that was the last time they appeared affectionately attached. Who knew then that it was their first and last warm get-together.

Divyansh's second-semester college examination was round the corner. He was in full steam with his preparation. Attending classes regularly, consulting teachers to make up the classes missed on account of intermittent travel to Jerusalem earlier and self-study became his daily routine. Amidst all this, he never forgot to punctuate his studies with writing poems and his reflection on his dedicated blog wall. For me, life seemed to be limping back to normalcy.

And then, yet another time!

Towards mid-February, Divyansh started complaining of headaches. Initially, I treated this as a one-off event and ignored it. But they kept coming. Despite this, Divyansh went to college regularly and kept his studies on. I became circumspect. The nature of his headaches seemed to have some sinister cause. Behind the facade of normalcy, I could sense a big danger lurking. The unsettling pain kept coming back to him after the effect of the pills wore off.

In 2005, we left Kolkata after Sushil was transferred to Mumbai. While we were in Kolkata, we used to visit the Kali temple in Dakshineshwar regularly. Before leaving for Mumbai, we went to the temple to seek her blessings. Unfortunately, we reached the temple late that day, and before we could reach the sanctum sanctorum, the door was closed. Left with no choice, we worshipped from outside and returned home. This had been haunting me since we came to Mumbai. Although I would try to dissuade myself of the irrational feeling that she didn't choose to bless my family on that day before leaving for Mumbai, I could never detach myself from this inconsolable thought. Whatever was happening to my son was slowly cementing this inexplicable perception. I asked Sushil if we could visit Dakshineshwar to beseech her forgiveness if I had done any wrong and to bless Divyansh with a healthy life.

We planned a one-day trip to Kolkata. We went to the Dakshineshwar Temple straight from the airport. I remember, that day, the queue at the temple was very long since it was some auspicious day. After nearly two hours in the queue, we reached her divine lap. There was such a rush that it was not possible to stay for more than 30 seconds there. In those 30 seconds, only tears of a helpless and hapless mother beseeched her forgiveness and sought blessings for her son. Divyansh. For a moment, I stopped feeling the constant shoving by the people around me. I became completely deaf to their screaming, hearing only the pristine sound of tears rolling down my face, which, perhaps, were the only offerings an ill-fated mother could give her that day. Before leaving the temple complex, I tied a thread to a sacred tree to fulfil my wish to see Divyansh free of all his miseries. It was said that whosoever wished for anything and tied a thread with that thought, it was granted, sooner or later. We returned to Mumbai on the same night with a profound feeling of redemption.

2

THE GUSH OF TYPHOON

My real understanding of Divyansh as a divine soul started when he was first diagnosed with leukaemia in December 2009, at the age of 12. I am not saying this as a mother. Others may take this as an exaggerated emotional outburst on my part; I won't fault them. Actually, when I join the dots of his life—before and after 2009—I find a certain symmetrical pattern in them. He was born to me with a purpose, which I started realizing only since December 2009. I conceived Divyansh in April–May of 1996. It was a difficult conception with intermittent complications. The doctor used to say that in the normal course of events, I would have lost him in the first trimester itself. But it seemed he was determined to be born to me. His ordeal continued even after his birth. He developed some serious medical problems after my C-section delivery. However, he recovered very fast from the temporarily scary situation. There was no looking back after that. It seemed he was in a tearing hurry to achieve everything for himself and to give joy and a sense of pride to the people he came across. The attending paediatrician always appeared to be in awe of his developmental milestones. In no time, as he grew, Divyansh became a darling, not only to my family and to our extended family but also to the neighbourhood in Kolkata where we lived at the time he was born. He started schooling and he adapted to the new environment in no time. Whenever I watched him sleep after toiling through the day, I would ride over the pinnacle of my motherhood. It always occurred to me that we both were made for each other. He had some inborn Midas touch, wherein whatever new things he tried, he excelled in, whether it was sports, music, writing, elocution, dancing or anything. He was a very fast learner. Since he was barely five years old, he developed an uncanny habit of communicating with us in writing. He would give small notes to me or to Sushil to express his emotions or if he wanted us to get him something.

One noticeable feature I had observed was that his writings, no matter how raw they were then, were always laden with truthfulness.

When he was barely five years old, one day, Sushil slapped him for something he had done wrong. Divyansh didn't show any emotion then. By evening, he gave a small scribbled note written in pencil to his papa, 'What did you get by beating me? Whatever you want to say, maybe in deep anger, can't you do that with love? *Agar maarna hi hai to scale se maariye, mere sar ke baal gusse me kyon khinchte hain?*' (If you want to beat, don't do that by pulling my hair. Use a ruler instead.)

Another note I am reminded of was the one he gave his papa on his promotion.

> Congratulations on your promotion. Now I will tell my books to be ready as there comes my best teacher, that's you, to teach me as you would be able to give me more time now. I promise, when I grow up, I will become a person like you and your name will be at the highest place.

Sometimes he would write letters to God to share his emotions. The integrity of his personality was something I was always proud of. After Sushil's transfer to Mumbai, Divyansh joined a new school in a new environment and adapted very fast. Apart from his excellence in extra-curricular activities, he was always one of the toppers of the class. I always waited for parent–teacher meetings at his school to drench myself in the ample praise for him from his teachers.

I distinctly remember that he gradually became quieter after the birth of my daughter Ananya in 2002 and even more so after 2005, when we came to Mumbai. Yes, I did notice it but never tried to get to the bottom of it. The real reason for this I could only fathom in December 2009.

Towards the latter half of 2009, Divyansh intermittently showed signs of some infections, followed by bouts of fever which subsided after medical intervention. When it happened for the third time in less than three months, and also noticing his significant weight loss, the attending paediatrician Dr Mukesh Sanklecha prescribed a series of tests. Test after test was done, and finally it was time for the last one—the bone marrow test. I was completely shaken. The test report hadn't come, but it seemed the oncologist was dead sure of what was coming to him. Could this happen to Divyansh? What have we done to deserve this? Divyansh was only 12 at that time. I was completely engulfed in such thoughts and apprehensions. Divyansh, on the other hand, blissfully enjoyed his favourite channels on TV with the remote in his hands laced with IV lines in the hospital.

The next morning, the doctor came into the room to see Divyansh and to inform us about the bone marrow test result. Sushil, apprehending something sinister, took him out of the room.

And we were crestfallen.

It was leukaemia, blood cancer—the deadly C that I had feared. I couldn't control myself. I don't know how many times I fell down after hearing this news. I cursed my fate; even questioned the existence of gods. I actually felt the re-joining of my umbilical cord with Divyansh and I experienced this C in me. When I looked at Sushil, I felt pity for him. It was a double whammy for him. On the one hand, his son had been diagnosed with cancer, and on the other hand, he had to control, pacify and counsel me. And then he had to deal with all the medical treatment issues. In the midst of it all, he had to appear cheerful to his son, as if nothing serious had happened to him. Where was the time left for him to cry in extreme pain, which he must have certainly felt? He seemed to have ingested his tears. He would meet the doctors, nurses and visitors with a smile on his face. Later, he confessed to me that he had found the strength to deal with this extreme hardship from none other than Divyansh himself.

The treatment was started by mid-December, to be precise, on 14 December. Divyansh never asked us what had happened to him. We never wanted to disclose the facts to him or utter the horrible C word. But even at the tender age of 12, he had a realization of what had befallen him and why he was undergoing such rigorous treatment processes. His hospital stay during that time was about a month. The treatment started, and true to his nature, every day before sleeping, he wrote in his diary with his hand punctured with IV lines. I was curious as to what he was writing. I didn't dare see his notes; he would never have wanted that. As the days progressed, my inquisitiveness to read his writings grew more and more. He started responding to the treatment very fast and achieved full remission within 10 days of the treatment. However, the treatment protocol was for two-and-a-half years, of which it was rigorous treatment for the first six months. One day, while he was writing before going to sleep, I told Divyansh about my desire to read his notes. He said, 'Mummy, you can read it tomorrow, as I will complete my write-up today.' It was difficult for me to wait for the next day to read all that he had written for himself in his tormenting hours. Did he know what had happened to him? The very idea used to make me shudder. I felt asphyxiated.

The next evening, after visiting hours were over, I caressed his forehead, kissed him, hugged him and asked about his notes.

He smilingly handed over his priceless diary, which is now my treasured belonging. The very title of his note ripped me apart. It read: 'The Time When I Was Closest to My Mother'.

I took a long pause before proceeding to read further. The daily notes of a boy, merely 12 years old, were long and, at one point, he had admitted that 'I am not completely graduated with hands to write about the care and compassion of my mother, yet I am trying to attempt it.' The note started with a question:

I am in the hospital undergoing treatment for some major medical problems. Christmas is round the corner. I was wondering, what will I do? Did Santa Claus have no surprise for me this year? But no, I was totally wrong. He did have a very big gift for me. Perhaps one of the best I have ever got up till now.

Divyansh knew that he was undergoing treatment for major medical problems, yet, he foresaw Santa Claus getting him the best gift of his life. He saw life, a brighter life amidst darkness all around. That was the first life-lesson I learnt from him that day. But what gift had Santa brought him, I still wondered. Then I read his thoughts in the subsequent pages, which cemented my belief in his indomitable spirit to live his life with zeal and zest.

He wrote:

I didn't get enough time from my mother after the birth of my sister, Ananya. She mostly used to be occupied with her as she was growing. But, when I was admitted to the hospital, now she pays almost 100 per cent attention to me, neglecting Ananya. She now comes to the hospital daily, feeds me, plays with me, talks to me the whole day and does all that which I relish. I think it is the first time in a millennium that she played with me after my early childhood. It was as if I was born again, and she was doing her job of a mother caressing her baby. How happy and

delighted I am now! THANK YOU SANTA FOR SUCH
A WONDERFUL GIFT.

That night I cried inconsolably. First, I realized that even in adverse
circumstances, the beauty of life can be traced. It was a lesson
to me. This realization from my son was one of the best gifts
Santa had brought me as well. Despite adversities, a tender son
was trying to lend a helping hand to his mother and keep her in
good stead. He took my motherhood to a different level, where
my own perspective about my life began to change. And second, I
now knew for sure why Divyansh had become quieter since 2005.

Divyansh was discharged from the hospital in the second
week of January 2010. For the next six months, he was on active
treatment in a day-care facility of the attending physician, many
a time once a week and sometimes twice a week. He responded
well to the treatment. As the days progressed, his energy levels
went up. Barring a couple of bad patches where he had to be
hospitalized, the treatment progressed well as per protocol. We
had an unspoken understanding at home that we would never
utter or discuss the C word. We only discussed the treatment
and a promising life beyond it. But at the end of the day, I must
admit, I lived in constant apprehension. I was psychologically
dented. No matter what lessons I had learnt from Divyansh, for
me, they were difficult to practise. There were people around me
who always discussed the nature of this life-threatening disease.
Such people unsettled me. They were the ones I always prayed
should not visit. Such people, no matter how good their intentions,
left a convulsive sensation in me. Some would talk only about
cancer, which would stir me with unsettling fear and pain. I
often felt like shouting at them, and saying, 'Please leave me. Be
sensitive to a vulnerable mother.'

One of my close relatives stopped bringing her sons to our
house, apparently to shield them from my son, fearing the bad
spell of cancer might cast a shadow on them too. I distinctly

remember that some of my neighbours would stop their children from entering the elevator when Divyansh was inside.

Yes, there were some people who avoided such discussions, and talked about subjects which I liked. During those times, there were people, some of whom were my own relatives, who often said, 'Nidhi doesn't want to meet anyone. She doesn't want to talk.' Such people never tried to understand why I did that. I was gradually being alienated. They seemed to have started deserting me; their alibi was that I was the reason for that. They could not even touch the periphery of my mental agony and fathom my predicament.

As for Divyansh, he was just the opposite. At such a tender age, circumstances led him to walk on the edge of a razor, yet he was well composed while facing gusty winds. He never appeared vulnerable to me as his mind had firmly controlled any panic. He never liked to discuss his day-to-day medical problems and always tried to keep them to himself. Sushil never allowed me to get involved in the treatment process. Perhaps he was mindful of the emotional vulnerability of a mother. Whenever I asked Divyansh about his medicines, he would say, 'Don't bother yourself, Mummy. I will take care.' He always made sure that he took his medicines himself and never allowed me to touch his medicine box. Ironically, how sensitive a 13-year-old boy was to his mother then, I realize now. Maybe, by doing all this, he was trying to heal the psychological dent I had suffered. In hindsight, I feel his sense of care for me, despite his suffering from extreme adversities, perhaps, outshone mine.

The six months of rigorous treatment period were over, and he was now all set to join his school in Class 8. For the next two years, he had to go to the day-care facility once a month for maintenance therapy. At this juncture, I must mention the name of Ms Alice Carvalho, the then principal of St. Mary's School, where Divyansh was a student. He had to miss the final term examination because of his medical problem. Nevertheless, she thought it fit to promote him to the next class. All through his stay in school, Ms Carvalho used to take care of him personally. Sushil shared with me his experience when Divyansh went to school for the first time after seven months of lay-off. Donning the white school uniform and a black skull cap, when Divyansh stepped onto the paved narrow strip leading to the assembly hall, he looked a bit shaky. Sushil wondered what must have been going on in Divyansh's mind when he would face his peers and teachers after a long time. Actually, they knew what had happened to him. And the skull cap is always testimony of a person just coming out of treatment for cancer. Sushil said that just before entering the assembly, Divyansh had looked up the sky for a moment, and then, with complete elan, walked inside the assembly hall. Sushil couldn't hold his tears. It seemed his tears were accustomed to seeing the world when no one was around. He was at the school gate at exactly 3 p.m. to receive him, that being his first day after lay-off. The way Divyansh came out of school after the last bell rang for the day, it seemed he had completely dwarfed his absence of seven long months of his tumultuous life. Thank you, Ms Carvalho, for being a good samaritan for my son when it mattered the most to him.

Divyansh grew his friendships in a new way in school. In Delzad's words, they were the Three Musketeers, Athos, Porthos and Aramis: Divyansh, Rao and Delzad, respectively. Athos was the wise leader, the enlightened one. Porthos was the motley one and Aramis was the ambitious one. Talking about homework one day, Divyansh noticed Delzad sulking all day but he stayed silent and let him have his space. Delzad finally gave in and told him about his heartbreak and brought it up repeatedly, despite the other two trying to soothe his mood. Eventually, Divyansh lost his cool, narrowed his eyes, pointed all five fingers at him and shouted, '*Ay! Jo ho gaya so ho gaya na … Jo nai hua woh kar!*'

(Whatever is done is done … Focus on what is left!). Delzad asked, '*Kya nai hua?*' (What is left to be done?). Divyansh lightened up with a smirk and said, 'Your Hindi homework.' They laughed and gossiped and, of course, finished their homework just in time.

Divyansh was a humble and respectful person, but he wouldn't let others make fun of him. There is an incident to justify that statement. Once, Divyansh, after coming back from school, told me, 'It was a noisy classroom and we were seated near the window. I was chosen to stand and recite a verse from the textbook to the class. Halfway into the verse, Sir cut me off and told me, "Speak louder yaar! Your words are flying out of the window." Wittily, I came up with a comeback. I moved around my desk, went to the window and started shutting all the windows one by one. There was an eerie silence in the class as they all watched me closing all the windows of the classroom. Then, without any expression, I came back to my place and asked Sir, "Better?" The whole class laughed, cheered and clapped for me. Sir himself gave a cheery smile and laughed, asking me to sit.'

With time, I also regained my emotional groove and started participating in the social life around me. The nightmare of Divyansh's medical problems still rumbled inside me. For his healthy life, from that very year onwards, I began to perform Chhath Puja when I was still in my 30s. This festival is celebrated with utmost reverence in North India, more specifically in the states of Bihar, Jharkhand and Uttar Pradesh. The Chhath Puja is dedicated to the Sun and Chhathi Maiya to thank them for bestowing bounties of life on earth and with a desire to enable the granting of certain wishes. The person who observes the Chhath ritual is called Parvaitin, and has to fast for three days and lead a restricted life during those three days. Whenever I used to offer Argha to the setting and rising Sun God, I would only wish him to build a castle around Divyansh to protect him from bad spells. Our lives seemed to have now fallen in place.

Divyansh was shining at school and became the blue-eyed boy of all his teachers. His academics were superlative and he consistently remained one of the toppers of his class. It became a regular feature for him to collect awards and accolades on the School Annual Day. I quietly nurtured my desire to see him collecting the award for the best student after he completed his Class 10 board examination. Whenever I discussed it, Divyansh would only give me a gentle smile. I didn't know what his smile meant then. That was for a purpose which I realized a couple of years later. Divyansh, by that time, joined a cricket academy under a coach named Mr Parandkar, who started grooming him for fast bowling. He represented his class in the school cricket matches and became known for his immaculate fast bowling skill. Sushil now was completely immersed in his office work. Ananya had also regained her emotional balance. We were fast galloping towards a normal life, forgetting the dreaded event as a bad dream.

Could this normalcy sustain?

3

HALFWAY DOWN THE PATH NOT UNTAKEN

March 2012.

Divyansh was back from school after finishing his last paper of the final term of Class 9. He had done exceedingly well in all papers and was all set to begin his final year of school starting in June. His maintenance treatment was also due to get over by May. I heaved sighs of relief as Divyansh approached the end of the treatment protocol. The attending doctor was satisfied with his progress. Considering his upcoming two months of recess and the schedule of private tuitions for the board examination early next year, we planned a short trip to New Delhi to visit my younger sister Shikha and her family. For Divyansh, Shikha was another mother. He was affectionately attached to her. After staying with her for a week, we organized a family visit to Mathura, Vrindavan and Agra. Divyansh, for the first time, saw the Taj Mahal, the epitome of beauty of love and one of the Seven Wonders of the World. We were thoroughly fascinated to see the devotees of Krishna in Mathura and Vrindavan, completely mad in their Ras Lila. It was a perfect retreat for Divyansh and Ananya. However, towards the end of the trip, Divyansh looked a little spent and drawn. We thought it might be due to the fatigue caused by continuous travel.

Divyansh started complaining of intermittent headaches

without any other physical symptoms. Initially, we just treated it with standard analgesics.

I never imagined in my wildest dreams that what we were thinking would end by the next month was going to start once again.

In May 2012, when Divyansh was to start Class 10, the doctor informed us that the disease had relapsed in the central nervous system (CNS relapse). I was shell-shocked. It took me a few days to comprehend what CNS relapse meant and its implications on the ongoing treatment process. Sushil was mute, with a blank face, still trying to fathom the roads ahead. It was painful for me to digest the recurrence of the disease when the treatment process was just about to end and Divyansh seemed to have fully recovered, barring the headaches during the last month. Divyansh had followed his treatment protocol so assiduously that I felt wretched to have to accept this fate. It seemed like someone had stabbed Divyansh in the back when he had taken his life-challenges head-on and moved on with utmost poise and spirit. He was being quoted in his school as the quintessential person who had shown mental fortitude in the face of extreme adversities. As for me, at one point, I felt like losing myself. But then, I thought about Divyansh. How would he take this news? Now, he was relatively grown up. How would I face him? I was flustered with all these questions. Except for his physical discomfort, the mere gaze of Divyansh still consoled me. It seemed he wanted to say, 'Mummy, this too shall pass.'

The CNS relapse did not shatter Divyansh. The only regret he showed was that he was going to miss his school and crucial studies for the board examination. For the next two-and-a-half months, he remained in the hospital, undergoing chemotherapy sessions and struggling with multiple infections and the side effects caused by them. The relapse of leukaemia entailed more intense chemo sessions. More intense chemo sessions meant more side effects and low immunity. By mid-August, he was discharged from the hospital with the advice to undergo chemo sessions twice a week in the same day-care facility for the next two years. His dream of initiating Class 10 with high spirits and taking the board examination early next year looked shattered, at least to me. I felt cheated. The doctor advised him not to go to the school in view of his low immunity, which could expose him to infections. Besides, periodic chemo sessions were surely going to impede his regular studies. The Class 10 board examination looked like a distant dream. The doctor's opinion was to forget the examination and focus on what was most important then: the life-saving treatment.

But Divyansh was determined and steadfast like the Rock of Gibraltar. He asked his father and me to permit him to prepare for the board exams from home. That was the last week of August. By that time, he hadn't attended school for even a single day. Also, going by the doctor's advice, he could not attend school in the coming days as well. But considering his determination, we encouraged him to prepare from home. I thought the studies would keep him in the right spirit while taking treatment. However, I had some doubts that he would be able to even complete his studies, forget appear for the exams. Divyansh started preparing for the exams from home and, many a time, from the day-care centre where he underwent treatment. For the next six months, Sushil became his teacher and a student as well. A student, because he would go to Divyansh's school to meet his teachers every day to take updates on the progress of various subjects. Those were not the days of WhatsApp. I did what I could do to take care of even his minutest needs and generally tried to keep him in good cheer. My heart would rip apart seeing him study in extreme physical discomfort. Whenever I saw the other children of my colony in school uniform going to school, rather than feel bad for my son, I felt proud of him, at the way he was earning his studies. His determination to move on in life was something I would cherish all my life. It really required colossal efforts to study while undergoing treatment, with severe side effects and exacerbating physical and mental conditions. There was another collateral problem he faced, which he never allowed to surface on his face. As he was away from his school, his friends were slowly drifting apart. The importance of friends, especially in critical times, can't be overemphasized. One goes and the other steps in. In these crucial times, his cousins Mridul and Anshoo became his friends, maybe more than that. It was timely relief for me to see their captivating bond when it was required the most.

Finally, the day arrived when he went to appear for the examination without attending even a single day of school. Alongside the exams, he was taking treatment as well. I prayed for him to at least finish his exams, no matter how he performed. He had painstakingly studied hard in poor physical conditions. Academic results were of no meaning to me. He was appearing for a bigger examination in his life, where merely attempting to appear in these circumstances was considered a success.

I, overawed by his academic excellence, always dreamt, like any mother would, that a day would come when he would go the dais of the school stage to collect an award for being the topper in the board examination and would get a standing ovation from one and all present there. However, after the relapse of the disease and the medical conditions in which he was studying thereafter, I felt devastated and stopped nurturing this dream.

Finally, the board exam results were announced, in May 2013. He scored 94 per cent and stood sixth in the school. Honestly, I never expected he would give such a stupendous performance, considering his adverse surrounding circumstances. I had just prayed that he would pass out along with his peer group. Sushil, normally a man who held on to his nerves in such situations, texted a message to Divyansh:

I had read a quote of Ralph Waldo Emerson written near the gates of the principal's office in your school: 'What lies behind you and what lies in front of you pales in comparison to what lies inside you.'

Divyansh, you epitomize this thought. I feel too small to even congratulate you on your stunning success. Let me, nevertheless, congratulate you on possessing and harnessing this formidable force inside you and showing us the way to move forward in our lives. To me, you have topped the examination of life. Now I realize that right from December 2009, when you were first diagnosed with C, rather than us guiding you, you have been guiding us to tread against the gusty wind. I am blessed to be your father. God bless you.

When Divyansh showed me this message, I could not have agreed more with Sushil. What he gave was a new boost to my sagging self-belief. It was as if I had reached an oasis in a desert. Here again, he lent his helping hand to a sulking mother, as before.

Mother's Day was round the corner. Divyansh, in his classic style, gave me a long letter to celebrate motherhood. The opening para of the letter gave me the first glimpse of the divine design of why he came into my life. I am still clueless about what made him write like this. It read:

12 May 2013

One day, Lord Brahma was sitting on his throne, looking very pensive. All the planets and stars were revolving around him. Just then, Lord Shiva came by. He asked him, 'Oh Great One! What is worrying you?' Lord Brahma replied, 'As the Creator, I have to send a child to Earth, into a woman's womb. This child might face some problems in his formative years. Hence, I need a mother, who is capable enough to raise this child holistically, stand against all odds for the child, has the ability to sacrifice and love at the same time and act as a shield for the child. I have not yet found any woman capable of all this.' Just then, Goddess Parvati came there, searching for Lord Shiva. When she heard all this, she said, 'Don't worry, I will send a part of my motherhood soul with this child in her. She is fully capable of all this. She will be the incarnation of my motherhood.'

Thus, dear Mummy, you were chosen to be my mother. And maybe that is how my name became 'Divyansh'.

The letter further said:

Let me tell you, Mummy, I absolutely love spending time with you. There are no barriers; I just feel so comfortable and positive around you. I am at peace with my surroundings and with myself, which one experiences through prayers and in God's presence. Your smile and laughter are the most beautiful spectacles for me. You truly are the incarnation of Goddess Parvati: a mother who can do anything for her children. They say that parents are the second form of God. But I believe you to be my primary God.

Interestingly, he ended the letter with a disclaimer, which read:

This story is a work of my imagination to showcase your greatness.

I still wonder: was it mere imagination or done for some mediated purpose?

It was the fag end of June. Sushil got a call from Divyansh's school to attend the upcoming award function along with Divyansh. I wondered what award he would get. We attended the award function in July. The principal of the school, Father Misquitta, after his initial presentation on the academic year 2012–13, announced the school toppers of the board examination. He named the first five toppers. And then, he paused, and invited the attention of all those present there to a PowerPoint presentation on Divyansh Atman, acknowledging his grand success in the face of acute adversities, and this, without attending school even for a single day. As the presentation on him was going on, my heart began beating very fast. It seemed something unexpected was going to happen. The principal then announced that the school, from that very year onwards, had instituted an award named The St. Mary's School Special Award despite Some Form of Disability, and Divyansh Atman became the first recipient of this award. When Divyansh went to collect his award on the dais, he got a roaring standing ovation from one and all till he went back to his seat after collecting the award. There were only two persons sitting on their chairs whilst others were standing and clapping. Paradoxically, they were me and Sushil. We were awestruck. We were completely clueless as to how to react. Quickly, I realized that my dress was getting wet with my copious tears and people sitting close to me were noticing it. Actually, they were hardly perturbed by my tears as some of them themselves had tears in their eyes. They were, at that moment, looking at the parents of an extraordinary person with a sense of amazement. I was quickly reminded of my dream to see him receive an award for the best student and his answering measured smile every time I broached the subject to him. Now, I decoded what his smile had then meant. He gave me much more than I had expected. Actually, on that day, Divaynsh Atman made his distinctive mark amongst others in the function, which was earned by dint of sheer determination and hard work. That day, I learnt another lesson of life: never ever lose hope. This was how Divyansh realized my dream, though in a different and an epic way.

His cousin Mridul had also attended the award function that day with us. He too couldn't control himself about what he saw happening before his eyes. After the function, he texted Divyansh:

I was sitting dumbfounded in the auditorium while basking in that momentous occasion. Amidst the thunderous applause, amidst tears of joy, some held back in humility, some brimming and overflowing, amidst choked hearts and hands held, amidst proud teachers and an audience left in wonder, you did it! You put us on the podium. Having seen you work for all this from close quarters and what has gone behind it to achieve this, I know. So, I can't begin to tell you how proud I felt to see the kind of reaction the audience gave your efforts. It was undoubtedly an experience of my lifetime. Congratulations!

Truly, as Tim Fargo said, 'Until you cross the bridge of your insecurities, you can't begin to explore your possibilities.'

Divyansh was ready for admission in a college. When I asked him about his future career options, I was amazed at his reply. After finishing junior college, he wanted to try for admission in MIT, USA, and pursue Computer Science. Honestly, when he spoke about it, I didn't even know the name of this university and what iconic value it carried. When he told me about it, I could only admire his spirit to aspire to study in this prestigious university despite the extreme adversities he was in. I was moved to see that he had masked his physical discomfort so successfully that it could not even touch his effervescent spirit to move on with his life. Actually, along with him, I was growing too; rather, he was helping me grow. His dreams were becoming mine. Here again, he was lending his mind to a mother to dream big.

Divyansh took admission in KC College, Mumbai, in the science stream. Now, his daily drill had begun. Attending classes in college, periodic, twice a week treatment sessions in the day-care centre and also attending coaching classes to prepare for the entrance tests for engineering colleges. It seemed too much for him and for me as well. Apart from that, one more issue was bothering me. Divyansh was now a 16-year-old youth. Normally, in the annals of one's life's journey, the beginning of college days carries a special meaning. We get to engage with a new band of friends. The atmosphere is more informal as compared to school. The level of interactions between them resonates the onset of youth in them. The treatment process Divyansh was subject to and its side effects had taken a toll on his body. He became overweight and there were other collateral effects that masked his physical persona. As a fledgling youth, he seemed well aware of his limitations in interacting with boys and girls of the college with all that was happening to him. As a mother, I always wished that my son should enjoy his life in college in the manner he wanted. Divyansh never stayed back in college after classes. I often wondered if maybe in the leisure periods, he was sitting somewhere alone or reading books in the library and not spending time with friends and enjoying carefree times as other youngsters did. Although Divyansh never let me know about this deprivation, I was sensible enough to read it from his face, though I might have been wrong in making this inference about him. Either way, Divyansh was not getting the kind of college life which he should have had. It was too depressing for me. Years later, one of his friends, Dhruv, wrote an email to Sushil where he articulated an observation about Divyansh that ripped apart my heart. He wrote:

> One of the bonds which I will forever share with Divyansh is that we were both battling cancer. A lot of people do not realize this but for a young boy, losing his hair can be a source of great discomfort. Though a lot of people may brush aside this concern, as another young man in the same predicament, I can assure you that it is a legitimate concern. This concern can fester if left unengaged.
>
> A few short years had passed since our first meeting at St. Mary's. Divyansh had visited my house with you. He was in his mid-teens and like many boys his age, he too was concerned about his looks. He had asked if it was still possible to meet girls and be romantically involved with

them given the lack of hair. This was a very understandable concern as I too had faced similar insecurities. I had assured him that many girls would love to meet him, as a hairline was not the only concern of women in our age group. It was important to be able to work on a talent to differentiate yourself from a crowd.

So, work on a talent to differentiate yourself from a crowd: was that so easy in the predicament Divyansh was in? Divyansh was determined to do it, yes, but it was difficult. His life had taught him a lesson to bring out the best in the most difficult situations. He had proved this in the past. Why not again?

The absence of one thing sometimes leads you to explore the presence of some other new things in and around you. That was the time Divyansh did two new things for himself: one at my own initiative and the other at his. I was very regular in yoga sessions conducted in my apartment complex by an accomplished and very nice lady, Mrs Raji. Through me and others, she had heard about the exemplary life journey of Divyansh and his achievements. Incidentally, her residence was just next to Divyansh's college. I thought a regular yoga session with her at her home would surely benefit Divyansh mentally and physically. Raji Madam instantly accepted my request to work with him after college hours. Divyansh, initially reluctant, agreed eventually to go to her. When I took him to Raji Madam's home for the first time, she later revealed to me that she fell in motherly love with Divyansh at first glimpse. And thereon began her poignant relationship with him, where she called Divyansh 'Hanuman', as his actions were like him. I heaved a sigh of relief to see Divyansh's daily physical and mental toll receive the spiritual balm of Raji Madam. Undoubtedly, Divyansh benefited a lot from her sessions. Raji Madam always showered her unconditional love and affection on Divyansh. Once Divyansh wrote a letter to her in which he philosophically articulated, 'I believe that

God is on everyone's side. It's just that we have to find him on our side and inside us.'

Raji Madam's reply was equally fascinating. She wrote: 'My one-faced little Hanuman, your letter to me is the most precious gift I have ever had in 63 years of my life. You will be my victorious Hanuman till my last breath.'

Raji Madam was always by his side in his best times, and more importantly, the most turbulent times, like a God, as envisaged by Divyansh.

The other new thing which Divyansh started on his own initiative was learning to play the guitar. He had an innate musical prodigy in him. In his childhood, he had learnt Hindustani classical music from Mr Vijay Prabhakar Thomre in Mumbai. But the catastrophe of December 2009 derailed his progress. Now, he wanted to continue his musical sojourn with a new shade. Savio, his guitar teacher, came into his life to reverberate his soul first with strings of the acoustic guitar, and later, the bass guitar. Savio was an extraordinary guitarist with a flair for teaching the finer nuances of strumming the strings. Besides this, what brought Divyansh very close to him, beyond the realm of the teacher–student relationship, was Savio's superlative humane touch when he spoke. They bonded so well that sometimes I was tempted to attend their sessions. Savio, more than playing strings, taught him the importance of music in life. Divyansh perhaps needed this the most then, who knew? Not me, at least. Perhaps he knew.

Ms Rati Dady Wadia was the ex-principal of Queen Mary School, Mumbai, who had retired in 2002. When Divyansh was due to appear for his Class 10 board exams, someone had recommended her name for English tuitions for him. Initially, considering her age, she was reluctant to take on his tuitions, but when Sushil narrated Divyansh's life journey and resolve to appear at the board examination against extreme adversities, she instantly agreed to help him better his language skills. Ms Wadia taught him English only for about two months before the examination. Two months of tuitions translated into a life-long relationship with him, and with us, way beyond Divyansh's own life in this world. As Divyansh would tell me, Ms Wadia taught him some of the finer aspects of English language which only she could have. She inculcated in him a value to use a language with utmost respect in whatever form of expression he wished. She also talked about the nine legacies of life which her late father practised. These were: love, truthfulness, contentment, dignity of human beings, to be happy under all circumstances, reliability, value for money, independence and unflinching faith in the Almighty. She would often tell Divyansh that he was one of the few students she had taught who practised all these nine virtues. Thus, the values inculcated by her went a long way in shaping Divyansh's literary journey in the later years of his life.

Another thing I absolutely must mention is that Divyansh began to read books in a big way after his relapse in 2012. He read a sizeable number of books of various genres like fiction, non-fiction, science-fiction, epics, drama, mythology, etc. in a short period. On his shelf, Dan Brown rubbed shoulder with the likes of Amish Tripathi, Mario Puzo and Khalid Hosseini, while Jawaharlal Nehru's *Discovery of India* competed with the Mahabharata, *The Hobbit* and *Harry Potter*. He would finish a bulky book so fast, it dumbfounded me.

Around that time, Divyansh also began to take great interest in understanding the finer nuances of culinary skills. He became a regular viewer of the show MasterChef Australia and its Indian version as well. In a short time, he became a huge reservoir of information on exquisite dishes apart from Indian foods. Once Mridul told me, 'I was amazed all the time because Divyansh has not ever been in a kitchen. But when we ate and there was something off, he could pinpoint exactly what was missing or wrong. Once, we were eating palak paneer at a restaurant and he was able to tell exactly which spice was too much and how the palak was just that much undercooked.'

I must confess, whatever cooking skills I possess should be greatly attributed to him. His reviews, in layers, of the dishes I prepared for him always motivated me to better my cooking skills. Every sincere cook craves for the perfect person to appreciate his/her cooking and give a genuine review. Divyansh was the one for me. He taught me the difference between a cook and a chef. He gradually shaped me into the mould of a chef from a cook. There was one similarity between us. Whenever I was stressed and finding it difficult to manage, I would go into the kitchen and prepare some special dishes for Divyansh and my family. It acted as a great stress-buster for me. Likewise, Divyansh had similar ways of managing his stress. He would be really pleased after savouring those stress-busting creations. There was a unique commonality of stress between us, which necessitated such dishes for its banishment. On my birthday, 14 July 2013, Divyansh had written a letter to me where he talked about it. He wrote: 'The best part about your great cooking skill is that you improvise and put perfection on a plate. If you make me do a blind tasting of a 100 dishes and ask me to identify which one was yours, I would not take more than a split second to do so.'

To me, Divyansh's life became an exemplary display that juxtaposed the extreme physical adversities he faced on account of medical problems with life-enabling virtues he learnt and possessed alongside. It felt to me that he was constantly subjected to a Samudra Manthan (Churning of the Ocean) where he himself swallowed all forms of poisons in his life and churned out Amrit (divine manna) for others to drink of.

So, amidst routine college classes and arduous medical treatment and its side effects, Divyansh, in parallel, started a spiritual and yogic journey with Raji Madam, the resumption of his musical sojourn with Savio and his own enlightenment through reading books. Ms Wadia had already taught him the importance of language in one's life. All these together propelled him to herald a new journey in his life: that of writing poems. He always reinvented himself. He now began to reinvent himself in a new way with a literary paradigm of his life.

Though Divyansh's soul always dwelt in me, the fact was that his ideal was his father, Sushil. He used to simply idolize him. Divyansh, silently, over a period of time, learnt from Sushil the art of perfection: be it lifestyle or managing household, office work or any work for that matter. His immaculate sense of dressing always fascinated him. Above all, the kind of management skills Sushil had exhibited with utmost poise when Divyansh was struggling on all counts, without compromising on official, familial and social responsibilities, was a virtue Divyansh always aspired to emulate. Divyansh's first forays into his literary paradigm were for his idol, his father.

He wrote the first poem of his life on 15 July 2014, titled 'His Name Personifies Him'.

When someone writes about his idol, it is usually a long précis or a poem. So was this poem of Divyansh. The following excerpt of this poem sum up the virtues Sushil possessed and which Divyansh adored.

> As someone who lives,
> Under the aegis of his shadows,
> Always protected, always carefree,
> Idolizing him, deifying him,
> I, my friend, have lots to say about him,
> Yet, I am speechless.

When Divyansh showed me this poem to comment on, I was completely amazed to see his skill of articulation, and his understanding and appreciation of his father. However, I distinctly remember Sushil felt embarrassed to read this poem, though he appreciated succinctly the beginning of Divyansh's literary journey.

Divyansh shared a special relationship with Mridul and Anshoo. Mridul was always by his side when the tides were against him. In those days, Mridul was working in Singapore and later shifted to Dubai. There was not a single day that Mridul did not talk to Divyansh on the phone. The exhilaration I witnessed when Divyansh talked to Mridul was soothing to me. They were more than brothers. Their camaraderie transcended the domain of brothers, their relationship appeared ethereal. Since my wedding, when Mridul had just stepped into his teens, I had seen him grow, and admired him a lot. Somewhere deep in my heart, I wished to see Divyansh become like him. So, to me, their growing chemistry always let me conjure Divyansh in Mridul and Mridul in Divyansh. However, later on in life, as I write his memoir, I realize how wrong I was then. Divyansh, as time progressed, started reflecting his own distinctive persona, and the differences in his ways of dealing with issues in his own life and those of others were monumental. I could see in him the seamless integration of the Eight-Fold Path of Life preached by the Buddha, leading to salvation. He led his life by example and his own mother began to emulate him in many aspects of her life.

Obviously, failing to attend the wedding of Mridul and Mahima in February that year due to medical treatment was a great disappointment to Divyansh. I am sure it was for Mridul as well. It gave me a nagging feeling of remorse about not being able to take him to Patna for his wedding. He may have wanted to go but respected my sentiments. On our return to Mumbai, I had something in my mind when I requested Mridul and Mahima to plan a trip to Mumbai. They did come later in the year. The feeling of ecstasy was palpable on Divyansh's face. We organized a small reception in Mumbai on 12 September 2014 to celebrate their wedding with all fun and frolic, where most of our friends attended with their families. The party was exactly as we had planned. Everyone danced, including Divyansh. I saw Divyansh dance after a long, long time. And I also danced with him perhaps for the first and, sadly, for the last time. That day I danced only for Divyansh. That was my way of bringing the joy of Mridul's wedding to him that he had to miss. Divyansh was worthy of this redemption.

His longing to meet his pal and his equally vibrant wife, Mahima, grew more with the passage of time. They had settled in Dubai and were busy in their own lives. Anshoo had also shifted his base to Delhi where he was struggling to manoeuvre his formative years of corporate life. Divyansh was again left alone with his nemesis. One of the Eight-Fold Paths preached by Buddha is 'Right Mindfulness'. That's what he practised here again.

One morning, I saw Divyansh in a thoughtful mood. I asked him about it. He said nothing. After breakfast, I saw him typing a poem titled 'The Ecstasy of Expectation', where he poignantly expressed his sublime imagination, where the apparent dream of meeting his buddy metamorphosed into reality.

Here is an excerpt of this poem, which Divyansh had written on 4 August 2014:

I was in the stage of slumber,
When the mind is in the deepest realm of sleep,
When the mind usually conjures,
Dreams that are too strong to leave.

Ironically, my mind was completely blank,
Something that I did not quite realize,
Only to have this flash of epiphany.
An epiphany
Of a happy reunion.

The poem, to my mind, was a perfect ode to their relationship. I was sure the way Divyansh expressed his feelings through this poem had touched them, as they reciprocated in equal measure after having read it. However, I am not sure now if the intensity of feeling with which the poem was written has made a permanent abode in their lives. As I see it, the past seems to have shifted.

In the middle of his regular treatment, one day, Divyansh was returning from the day-care centre along with Sushil. He looked a bit pensive and Sushil observed him looking outside the window of the car, searching for some answer from a constituent of the cosmos he felt attached to. That was 12 August 2014. Gazing in the same direction where he was, he asked his father, 'How much more treatment is left to be taken?' Sushil consolingly replied, 'Divyansh, we are halfway through. Don't think too hard. Time flies.' Divyansh didn't ask any further questions. Sushil felt he was not able to answer him convincingly, and Divyansh must also have felt the predicament of his father so he chose to give a brief reply. He was not gazing outside with a blank face. Actually, his father had replied with the key word 'halfway', which was expanded by that constituent of the cosmos he was communicating with. By the time he reached home, his countenance had changed and he looked more relaxed and at peace with himself. It seemed like he had got the answer he was looking for. That night, he wrote the third poem of his life titled 'Halfway Down the Path Not Untaken', in less than two months of his literary journey. This poem he had written for himself, finding answers to all his questions, which only he could have given himself. His contemplative ode evoked a sense of wisdom not only in him, but also to us. He, through this poem, again lent a helping hand to us by letting us realize some of our own unanswered questions.

Here are some excerpts:

Unfathomable are the ways of God,
No, we cannot gaze it,
He is a whimsical artist,
Who sways His brush as He wishes.

I was about to plant my feet
On the lush, green track,
But I guess He had other plans for me,
For He chose to change my track.

...

Now, as I stand halfway down this path,
I have finally understood
The nature of adversities
As quoted by all.

...

You see, adversity is
A poison with its own antidote,
A thorn with its own red rose,
A mistake with its own moral lesson
That always makes you realize
Its profoundness at core.

When I read this poem, its profoundness hit my conscience. He made me realize the purpose of my life, or rather, our lives, and its inner beauty. It was an epiphany that gave me a different perspective of all that was going on in our lives. Apparent may not be real, but the real must be actualized in us. That was my first peek at the idea that Divyansh had come into our lives with a purpose.

After Mridul and Mahima's reception, Divyansh was back to his own self and remained busy with his studies for the Class 12 board examination early next year, apart from the routine drill of his treatment. He gave a brief pause to his literary sojourn in order to focus on his studies. The next year, on 27 January, he would be 18 years old, an adult. He was quite excited about it. There were reasons for it. First, he would become eligible to vote in the elections. In his school days, he read and learnt the Constitution of India by heart. He always felt that the central theme of democracy was people's participation in forming governments. It was his long-cherished ideal to become a part of this process. Second, now he could watch A-rated movies. He had to miss some really good English movies just because they were rated 'A'. Sushil, Mridul and Anshoo would often tell him that he could watch them as those were rated 'A' for technical reasons in India, but he never did. He preferred to wait till he became eligible to watch them. He always practised 'Right Actions'. I distinctly remember the day he told me that the first thing he would do on turning 18 would be to watch one such classic 'A' rated movie that he couldn't see earlier. Third, as most of his friends were already on Facebook, he was eagerly waiting to turn 18 to be eligible to have a profile on this platform. The age restriction was one of the conditions of Facebook use in those days. He would not manipulate his age to start using Facebook earlier, like some of his friends had done. But fourth and most importantly, he was fed up of being addressed with 'Master' prefixing his name. The treatment process had become so protracted that in myriad doctors' prescriptions and tests reports, his name was always written as 'Master Divyansh Atman'. Those days were numbered now, after which he would be referred to as 'Mister' and not 'Master'. In fact, he told his father to give him a birthday cake, embossing his name on it as Mr Divyansh. So, we were all waiting for the day of his transformation from Master to Mr.

Would that be so easy?

Unlike our expectations, the New Year 2015 began with lot of challenges in Divyansh's life, and so, in ours too. Would some of my apprehensions come true? It seemed the Sword of Damocles was hanging over us. Divyansh again started showing symptoms of headache without any visible reasons. I thought that since his treatment was still in progress, there was no question of the disease returning. The doctor always gave a guarded response. Divyansh's eighteenth birthday was at hand. More importantly, I was tense about his board examination, beginning the next month. Divyansh had prepared against the backdrop of extreme physical and mental hardships. Like I said earlier, he had earned his studies all through the past months by dint of hard work. With all these anxieties brewing in my mind, we took an appointment with the doctor for the day after his birthday. We knew the doctor would possibly tell us something that could dampen the spirit of his celebration. Even though we were treading rough roads, we had to know the art of finding the best spots to plant our feet as we moved. Time had taught me this. More so, I learnt it from Divyansh. I was living my life in broken pieces. I had picked up one such piece to celebrate the heralding of his adulthood. We did our best to make that one of his wonderful days. But I knew, and perhaps more than me, Sushil knew, that the glass piece I had picked up to live my life to enjoy his birthday, was actually a glass shard which was ready to hurt me with its angular sharp edges.

The episodes of intermittent excruciating headaches remained unabated. A series of events led Divyansh to the ICU of a hospital in the first week of February. The board examination was to begin on 16 February. It now looked remote to me that he would be able to make it. A CSF test was done and the fluid was sent to another hospital for analysis and reporting. If the report read positive, it would be his second relapse of leukaemia. For me, accepting the likely news of a relapse was as painful as breaking it to my son and facing him since, so far, he had exhibited indomitable resolve to pace his life along with the treatment of the disease.

Since December 2009, when he was diagnosed with this disease, we never discussed it with him. We would normally discuss the treatment aspects but not the disease itself. There was an implicit understanding between us. I was aware that Divyansh knew that I never wished to broach the name of the disease before him. He also knew what he was suffering from. Yet, he respected my feelings by not taking the name of the disease before me. Equally heart-wrenching for me was to anticipate Sushil struggling to break the news to me and then trying to control my emotional eruptions. On the one hand, Sushil had to break the so-called shroud of secrecy of the disease to Divyansh, and on the other hand, he had to directly deal with a psychologically mutilated mother. How would he handle himself amidst all this? All these thoughts were playing on my mind. The report was to come in the evening. Some persons come into your life with a purpose. A couple of years back, Dr Archana Jadav, a CGHS doctor in Mumbai, had met Sushil when she came to see a patient in his office. I recalled then that her son had successfully undergone bone marrow transplantation (BMT) in Israel. By noon, Sushil called her and expressed his wish to meet her at her home to discuss the prospect of transplantation. She was aware of Divyansh's hospitalization and she immediately agreed to meet and help in whatever ways possible. Before the evening set in, Sushil broached the subject of transplantation to the treating doctor if the CSF report would come positive. He highly recommended this procedure. And so, before the report came in, we were ready with what we were up to and with a more enduring treatment option. When we are in the middle of a storm it's hard to think outside of it, but the only way out is to ride through it and hope that things will be a lot clearer on the other side.

The CSF report was delivered by 7 p.m. As expected, it showed malignant cells in the nervous system. It was saddening to us. But it didn't shake us, as we were ready to face another gusty wind with new armoury in hand. Sushil met Dr Archana in the evening who facilitated his talk with Dr Reuven Or, who had successfully treated her son in Jerusalem, Israel. Dr Or was a doctor of international repute and was a noble soul. Dr Archana encouraged Sushil to call him as he was quite an informal person and a religious Jew. As Sushil told me, that day was a Saturday and Dr Reuven was just done with Sabbath prayer when he spoke to him, in heavily Hebrew-accented English:

Mr Poddar, Sabbath Shalom. I am aware of your son's case.
Dr Archana has already briefed me about him. You please
mail me all his medical reports. I will do my best. Today
is Sabbath which is an auspicious day. I am just done with
the Sabbath prayers. Plan your trip to Jerusalem. You all
will be a part of my family. And please call me anytime
you need any advice or moral support as such. I am just
a call away.

It was like a dream for us to have been showered with such
comforting and reassuring words from someone of the stature
of Dr Reuven Or when we needed them the most. This infused
a new ray of hope in us.

Normally, people plan their visit to USA or to European
countries for the treatment of diseases like this. Honestly, this
thought did come to our minds. But after having talked to Dr
Or, I found a great degree of solace and, thus, gave this thought
a go-by.

The next day, Sushil met Divyansh in the ICU early in the
morning. Divyansh knew what was coming. Without too much
discussion of the reports and disease, Sushil straightway talked
about transplantation and the gist of his conversation with Dr
Or. Sometimes a parent searches for the shoulder of his/her son
to lean on. But not on those days, when the son himself requires
such support. We were lucky that day.

'Papa, let's finish it once and for all. Let's go for transplantation.
I am ready. You please chill,' Divyansh smilingly gave his verdict
and conscientiously broke the shroud of mystery of the disease
that we had created.

He, thus, once again allowed us to lean on his shoulder to
support us and lent a helping hand when it hugely mattered
to me.

Ananya was in Class 7 then. Her final examination was
soon to commence. Sushil suggested that I let him travel with

Divyansh for his treatment and that I should stay back in Mumbai to take care of Ananya. Theoretically, his advice at that juncture could not be debated. But just think from a mother's perspective! How could she allow her son to travel abroad to manage one of the toughest medical treatments? Won't he need gentle caresses, tight hugs and motherly care the most then? And how would I be able to breathe in his absence when my own breath would leave with him? I was being barraged with innumerable questions through which it was difficult for me to navigate. Equally difficult was for Divyansh to leave me and his adorable sister Ananya in Mumbai.

But Divyansh, as always, came to my rescue. He understood what was going on inside me. He hugged me and guided me to do what was most appropriate then. It is said that compromise is usually seen as a sign of weakness. Strong men never compromise. Not then. Divyansh and I compromised for better reasons and to gain strength in each other's absence. On the flip side, I wanted Divyansh to leave for Jerusalem, with or without me, at the earliest, not wasting any more time here. I thought he would be safest there, bringing his long journey of C to an end. His immediate travel held a lot of promise. I budged and allowed him to travel without me. He consoled Ananya by advising her to join him in Jerusalem when her summer vacations began after the exams. When he left Mumbai with Sushil, my heart went along with him. That was all I could do then.

Divyansh was due to appear at the board examination in February which he couldn't. In normal circumstances, I would have applied tilak on his forehead and wished him good luck. This opportunity came in a different way when he left for Jerusalem. I applied the tilak on his forehead with the same fervour and wished him good luck for a bigger examination in his life. The idea of redemption is always good, even if it means sacrifice or some difficult times.

Divyansh texted me as he was about to take off on 28 March 2015:

Mummy, please achche se rehna. Be strong. Ananya ke liye aur apne liye ekdum cheerful rehna. Aur apne aap ko engaged rakhna. Aur please rona mat. Apne aur Ananya ke sehat ka dhyan rakhna. Ananya ko kal walk pe le jaana. Kabhi kabhi restaurant bhi. Aur please achche se rehna. Ananya ko jyaada mat daatna. Love you mummy.

(Mummy, relax and be strong. Always be cheerful for Ananya and yourself. Keep yourself engaged. Take good care of your health. Take Ananya for a morning walk tomorrow. Sometimes take her to a restaurant also. Don't scold Ananya too much. Love you Mummy).

As he flew to the Holy Land to salvage his lost friend 'health', I was reminded of Divyansh's thought, beautifully penned in his poems:

> You see, adversity is
> A poison with its own antidote.

Bon voyage, Divyansh.
God bless you.

4

REBIRTH

You remember the day when a shard of glass ruthlessly pierced through your skin and sinew, badly bruising your right hand? And on top of it, you are a right-handed person. But even though the doctor advised you to rest, you carried on doing your daily chores undeterred. I was moved to tears seeing you cook, wash, dust, carry heavy bags etc. in such a condition...

After Divyansh left for Jerusalem with his father on 28 March 2015, the first thing I remembered was the concern he had shown when I had accidently cut my finger badly with a glass shard. He was so concerned that he even made a note about it in a letter on my next birthday.

I wondered if he thought about me and Ananya, and how I must be managing without him. The pain of my concern for him was getting compounded by the thought of his concern for me. He shouldn't worry about us—that was the first thought that flashed in my mind. I had to stay positive and reflect calmness to Divyansh whenever I talked to him: that's what I decided to do. But mere reflection was not sufficient if I didn't alter my own attitude to this effect.

Normally, at such times, my mother or younger sister would stay with us to lend helping hands and generally keep me in good spirits. But not this time. I decided to practise some sort of penance where I would reinvent myself and work on my attitude in order to make positive changes in me. I had seen Divyansh practise this many times. I made a tough decision and told my mother and sister not to come and stay with me this time. I am sure they questioned my decision to go along alone in the absence of Divyansh and Sushil. But the biggest factor that helped me manage my daily life alone was the feeling that Divyansh was now in a safe haven and his nagging medical problems of years would come to an end. As a matter of fact, even before Divyansh's actual treatment started in Jerusalem, I recouped my energy and redirected it to heal my wounds caused by years of his turbulent life. Ms Rati Wadia, Divyansh's English teacher, then came into my life as a healer. She invited me to her home twice a week and would engage me through her exposition on English literature and the importance of prayers.

When Sushil and Divyansh reached Jerusalem, the people of Israel were celebrating the festival of Passover. Jews celebrate this festival to commemorate the liberation of the 'children of Israel', who were led out of Egypt by Moses. I felt their arrival in Jerusalem couldn't have been better timed. Yes, it seemed the festival of Passover also had great significance for Divyansh and would liberate him from the clutches of his nemesis.

I had packed enough cooked food and groceries in their baggage when Divyansh and Sushil left for Jerusalem. But the cooked food couldn't have lasted long. It was not the questions of a few days. They had to stay there for months: how many, even the treating doctor did not know. Sushil, in all his life, had never cooked. He told me that the first dish he had prepared for Divyansh was khichdi and that was a disaster. He, instead of salt, had added sugar to it. That day, Divyansh was to be given light food as he was made to remain empty stomach all day long due to some procedure. When Divyansh started eating, he didn't utter a single word. He kept eating with utmost ease. Sushil expected some words of encouragement on his maiden venture in cooking, which would have propelled him to better his cooking skill. It didn't come. When he realized his blunder, he only lamented his apathy towards cooking food earlier in his life. He felt that since he had brought Divyansh thousands of miles away from his mother, it was his responsibility to bring some semblance of motherhood in him by taking care of his palate. Sushil expressed his concerns to me on the phone. We mutually discussed a solution.

An idea flashed instantly.

Each day before cooking, Sushil would tell me what he intended to cook and I would tell him on the phone how to cook that. Gradually, he became my sincere student, a student who used to apply my theoretical inputs to practice almost immediately, and would share the preparations on WhatsApp to get my approval before feeding Divyansh. My very approval on the digital platform was considered enough to render a motherly touch to the food that he prepared. The idea clicked. That way, Divyansh was served food which had loads of motherly flavour rendered through the sincere hands of his determined father.

Anshoo took leave from his office and joined them after a few days. The feeling that Divyansh now would have the company of his close pal Anshoo and Sushil would get help in cooking was comforting to me. It was very nice of Anshoo to take a month off from work since his was a new job then. I don't know how he managed it but I was grateful for it.

In the beginning, most of the establishments in Israel were closed for the Passover festival which lasted eight days, and the hospital where Dr Or was working was operating at the lowest staff capacity. So Dr Or suggested to Divyansh to visit important places in Israel. Anshoo, Divyansh and Sushil drew their travel itinerary meticulously so as to cover a maximum number of important places during the holiday. They first visited Bethlehem, the birth place of Jesus Christ; then Nazereth, where Jesus was said to have attained wisdom, and then travelled to the Sea of Galilee, which Jesus is said to have walked on. Finally, before embarking upon the treatment, they also visited the Old City of Jerusalem, where Jesus was crucified and was put to rest in a tomb. Divyansh knew what he had faced so far and what he was going to face required a new wisdom and perseverance, and he tried to absorb the spirit of Holy Land the most. He befriended a lot of Jews and they used to invite him on various religious occasions. He even attended Passover rituals in order to understand the deep-rooted meaning of it.

On 12 April 2015, Sushil called me to share the good news. That day they had gone to the hospital to meet Dr Or. For a BMT, the biggest challenge is to get a willing donor whose HLA typing of blood matches with those of the patients. It takes time. I was worried from day one whether Divyansh would find a donor and if he did, how much time it would take since they would have to stay there without any treatment for that period of time. To my immense relief, Dr Or shared the good news of a matching willing donor just after the Passover festival. When Sushil shared the news, my joy knew no bounds. I couldn't stop my tears, thinking that Divyansh was now a few steps closer to full recovery. What was left now was the actual procedure of transplantation. When I talked to Divyansh to share my joy about it, he gently spoke in a few words. I, as a mother, deciphered the ocean of his joy through each syllable of those few words. Perhaps those few words unwittingly conveyed to me a message to pack my bags and travel to Jerusalem to stand behind him when he would need me the most.

Preparing to go to Jerusalem to join our family, Ananya's joy was at a peak at the prospect of meeting her father and buddy Divyansh so soon. I was cognizant of two important issues concerning my personality, which would be put to test on this travel. The first issue was speaking English. I was born and brought up in a humble family where speaking even a single English word invited awe. I studied in a Hindi-medium school and even in college, the medium of instruction was mostly Hindi. When I got married to Sushil, he never considered not speaking English an issue. And why not, since Sushil himself had been brought up in a family where Hindi was the chief language of communication. While Divyansh studied in an English-medium school, his teachers coaxed us to speak to Divyansh in English so that he becomes proficient in the language. But even then, I never ventured to speak in English. Actually, this was never needed in my family. Had it been so, I would have picked it up early. I felt the first real need for this language when Divyansh began writing his poems. His English language was top class and, therefore, his poetry required a high level of language skill to comprehensively read and comment on. It was then on my mind to learn the language, and that's why, later, Ms Rati Wadia came in my life. A teacher who had taught my son was now all set to groom me to apply it meaningfully in my own life when I would need it the most. Considering this, I was mindful of having not-so-good communication skills in English, which would be required if I travelled abroad. To be fair to myself, I did have a fair exposure to the English language, but what was lacking in me was the self-confidence, which I now had to boost. For me, it was a small sweat considering the promise of meeting Divyansh and my husband soon.

Now for the second issue. While travelling, I was supposed to wear western attire, more specifically, jeans and a shirt or T-shirt. I was told that Israeli immigration authorities were quite particular while dealing with passengers looking like Muslims or those coming from Islamic countries. They would subject them to a higher degree of questioning. With my baby steps in speaking in English, I would have been thoroughly exposed answering their myriad questions as a result of the mere look of my dress.

In all my life, I had never worn jeans or western clothing. My traditional joint family upbringing clad me in salwar-kurtas or saris. Wearing jeans was considered taboo, at least in my family. Even after my wedding, I never gave it a try simply because I never felt like wearing it, though Sushil often nudged me to reconsider my decision. Now was the time for this reconsideration and unshackling myself from the do's and don't's of dresses that I had built around me.

Actually, there was also a third component attached to this thread. All my life I had never travelled alone. Before marriage, it was always with my parents, and after marriage, with Sushil. I never had the occasion to test myself through the procedural nitty-gritty at the airport. But I knew there wouldn't be problems on this count considering the passenger-friendly approach of the airline staff.

Honestly speaking, a part of all these predicaments of mine is attributed to Sushil. He was so caring that whenever we went out, it was he who used to command all affairs, saving me from the rigours of dealing with people when he was around. That's how he is. True to his nature, when Divyansh was diagnosed with leukaemia, he took everything on himself regarding his medical treatment, saving me from day-to-day hassles. However, later in our lives, when he felt it was my time to pitch in to handle his medical treatment, he quietly accepted it. He not only accepted it but appreciated me in no unequivocal terms. The way I handled all these issues came as a pleasant surprise to him. But that would be in the future, which I will talk about as I progress.

So, factoring these three issues, I was ready to embark upon my first solo journey and that too, abroad.

It was so relieving to meet Divyansh and my husband that it restored the feeling of my own existence. The family was reunited. I was geared to relieve Sushil from the bother of kitchen duties and the general upkeep of the apartment. But I realized that by that time, cooking had become a passion for Sushil. He would always insist on me allowing him to better his hands by cooking alongside.

My arrival in Jerusalem was timed to perfection. The actual treatment was soon to commence. I had heard a lot about the Wailing Wall of the Old City of Jerusalem. It's a holy place of the Jews where they lament the destruction of their temple and pray for its restoration. On a Sabbath Day, the ambience of this place was absorbing. Jews across all ages stand up along this wall and read the Torah. Besides, this place also draws teeming tourists who throng there for a feel of its magnificence. Visitors to the Wailing Wall follow the practice of putting small slips of papers upon which they write their prayers and wishes into the cracks between the stones. It is believed these wishes are granted. As Divyansh was to embark on a tough journey, I thought to pay a visit to this holy place before that. We visited the place on a Sabbath Day. What I saw there moved me. The atmosphere was electric. Sushil and Divyansh followed the local practice of wearing kippah before entering the wall premises. Ladies are not supposed to wear it. First, we washed our hands and then picked up small pieces of papers from the basket there. We each wrote our wishes and put them in the cracks of the wall. None of us spoke to each other about what we had written. We didn't even dare to ask each other for fear of risking the fruition of our wishes. It is said that eyes can't lie. When I looked at Sushil's eyes, I could decode that we had written the same wish. As for Divyansh, I never knew, though I was intrigued about it. I am still clueless about his wish that he had written on that piece of paper. As I write his story now, wisdom slowly permeates me which makes me feel that our wishes may not have been fulfilled on the face of it. However, a deeper understanding of the divine design gives a peek that this might have been fulfilled if we evaluate the subsequent events of Divyansh's and our lives from a different perspective. It is not a question of whether someone's wishes are fulfilled. On a higher pedestal of life, we must realize that what has to happen must and will happen. That is the ultimate fulfilment of our wishes. Who knows, the great Wailing Wall may have fulfilled our petitions kept in its core in a more majestic way. It is up to us how we look at it and assimilate.

Divyansh had suffered a lot since December 2009. Each and every day of his sufferings played before my eyes unabashedly. I was fed up with that. I always fancied giving him a new birth, a new life, free from what he had faced so far. I wanted to absorb the spirit of Mother Mary before giving him new birth in the holy land of Jerusalem. I was aware that it held great promise for his life. We, therefore, planned a visit to Bethlehem, where Mother Mary had given birth to Jesus Christ. I bowed with all my senses to the place where Mary gave birth to Jesus and prayed for her to bless me with her divinity for a new birth for my son. Jesus didn't live long but attained the most revered status of God. He had to suffer before attaining Godliness. Perhaps, Mother Mary had decided to give a new birth to my son through me to make him someone unique. Now, I realize what I didn't know then. Years later, whenever one of the greatest sculptures of all time, made by Michelangelo, in St. Peter's Basilica in the Vatican City, depicting the body of Jesus on the lap of Mother Mary after crucifixion flashes in my eyes, I get the same divine feeling of carrying my son on my lap. Bethlehem gave me new insight to nurture my motherhood to transcend the realm of life and death.

I don't know why, but the city of Jerusalem always gave me positive vibes. The structure and super-structure of the city are uniformly built with Jerusalem stones in a uniform shade of pale yellow all over. The city looked bright even on a cloudy day by the appearance of Jerusalem stones, which filled me with a gush of hope and energy. The people are divided between orthodox, semi-orthodox and unorthodox. Orthodox people always wear black suits, keep their hair long, wear black hats and read the Torah as per Jewish Law or Helakha. To me, they were easily identifiable by their attire. Semi-orthodox male Jews like Dr Or wear normal dress, but wear a kippah on their heads all the time and do not practise strict observances as followed by the orthodox Jews. However, they are very particular about the Jewish practice of observing Sabbath Day in accordance with its strict rules. Unorthodox Jews are those who do not even wear a kippah and generally seem to shun adherence to Jewish religious practices. They are the ones who are decried by the orthodox Jews for offending their religious laws and practices. Before my arrival in Jerusalem, Sushil and Divyansh had already befriended a lot of people, some of whom were Jews and some were Indians. The kind of comfort and help they extended to us remain permanently etched in my memory.

The availability of Indian groceries in Jerusalem had been a constant concern for me. Savdas, who was part of the Indian diaspora and is now a citizen of Israel, ran a grocery store in Tel Aviv, which was about 70 km from our apartment. He often dropped by at our apartment and supplied us with all the typical Indian groceries. That was a huge relief for us. He has a sweet family and his wife often invited us for dinner at their home. Navdeep Singh, another Indian who worked at the United Nations (UN) office in Jerusalem, was a pillar of support for us. He was ready to help us and was at our beck and call. It was he who had made the staying arrangement in an apartment and paid the advance when Sushil and Divyansh were planning to visit Jerusalem in March. Perhaps he had understood the pain of our long journey on troubled paths before we reached there. Though always on a tight office schedule, it never deterred him from visiting us regularly and helping us in whatever way he could. His sense of empathy for us and relentless hunger to lend us a helping hand reinforced my belief in the existence of humanity.

Like Savdas, he also often drove us to his home where his pretty wife Deepa cooked delicious food for us. Besides, we befriended a host of Jews, namely, Soshi, Caron, Jenny and her husband Zafi, Michell and Leuma and her husband Gideon. Here, it is apt to quote a few lines of a poem penned by Divyansh titled 'Rebirth', which was written after the transplantation, which I will discuss later:

A lot of inhabitants,
Who dwelled on the sidewalks,
Were my reliable guides,
Guiding me all the way.

As we were led on to tough paths in our lives by fate and time, these people were truly endowed with virtues that placed them high among the benefactors who constantly guided, comforted and unstintingly cleared our pathways as we walked ahead. Sushil has written reminiscences of some of these noble people, which you can read at the end of this book. Each and every word written by him about them is echoed by me with equal intensity.

On 10 May 2015, Mother's Day, Divyansh gave me a priceless gift while he was going through the greatest tribulation of his life. He penned a long poem for me titled 'The Tree of Purity'. Divyansh wrote poems in open verse and avoided writing in rhymes. He felt that open verse allowed him uninhibited expression whereas rhymes bound him. Each word of this poem spoke volumes on the profoundness of the mother–son relationship as he conjured. Not only his words but even the shadows of each line spoke aloud what he wanted to write but couldn't.

An excerpt is as follows:

She has let many of her branches break,
To let me grow uninterrupted, undisturbed from her,
With a base that is,
As strong and resilient as her.

> Mother, I promise you,
> As I grow longer and stronger,
> I will rise above and bend into the ground,
> To support you even stronger.

The underlying thought of the poem gave me courage to move on in my life amidst all adversities. In the worst of times, I always hoped that Divyansh would sooner or later rise to the occasion and support me as he promised.

Divyansh was mentally fully geared for the BMT. He started writing his experiences in the form of poems and articles as he went about the treatment process. A typical BMT had four phases. Phase I was the pre-transplantation phase, which involved a lot of tests and ablation chemo and radiation. This was done to kill your own body's cells and prepare it to receive the donor's cells. This phase spanned a month and a half. This was the phase where the patient's three main blood components, namely, haemoglobin, platelets and white blood cells, become almost zero, and this was the time when the patient was protected from infection in a quarantined environment. This phase, where your own body system was destroyed, was considered very painful. Phase II was the actual transfer of the donor's cells to the patient. Phase III was engraftment of the donor's cell in the patient's body. Then began Phase IV, which involved graft-vs-host disease (GvHD), which was again a painful stage where your own body cells recognized donor cells as the enemy and started attacking them.

I reached Jerusalem when radiation was due to commence. Divyansh tolerated the three-week long radiation sessions well. He had exhibited an uncanny knack of tolerating its side effects by constructively engaging himself in listening to his playlist. His favourite artists and bands that I could remember were Linkin Park, Coldplay, Justin Timberlake, Eric Clapton, Louis Armstrong, Pink Floyd, The Beatles, Bob Dylan and songs of Mohammad Rafi, and he had a special liking for albums of Niladri Kumar, especially *Plucked*. He went to the session with earplugs on and returned the same way. I was witness to what music therapy meant and how Divyansh was successfully able to handle the tormenting effects of radiation. The mind controls the body, but there are times when the mind needs to be controlled and that is done by our soul, which guides our mind to smoothly adapt to the changing physical conditions of the body. Divyansh had a good symbiotic connection between his mind and soul. The synergy between his mind and soul was on display for all of us to be inspired by. It was evident from the fact that when Divyansh began to experience hair fall due to radiation, he smilingly told me about his decision to go for a head shave. This was not the first instance of hair fall for him. It had happened many times back in Mumbai as a result of treatment, and every time it saddened me. I was reminded of the day when Divyansh had to get his head shaved again after the first relapse and I was hectically searching for his skull cap in my cupboard where I had hidden it from my sight once he was almost cured after the first bout of leukaemia. When I eventually found it, I was petrified to even look at it. The melancholic silence I felt after finding it was exasperating and I could not stop crying. But, over time, Divyansh had reconciled to the fact of occasional hair fall as a treatment hazard. I realized this due to his huge collection of caps of all hues and designs. His most favourite was a black one with a Roger Federer logo. Divyansh had made wearing caps his style statement. What a way to move on with his life! His spirit was inspirational. Deep in my heart, I still nurtured a desire to see him with a full-grown head of hair. He did eventually get his hair back in the last few months. Seeing it, I prayed to save it from evil eyes. But his hair fall this time didn't leave me feeling exasperated. I smilingly endorsed his decision. Perhaps that happened because I foresaw a brighter future for him after the transplantation, and so, the sight of hair fall and shaving didn't affect my mental condition.

Divyansh was finally hospitalized for transplantation towards the end of May 2015. As a part of Phase I, he still had to undergo ablation chemo. Dr Avni Batia informed Sushil about the adverse effect of ablation chemo on the fertility of patients. She was of the view that chemotherapy in general reduces the fertility of patients. Ablation chemo would do more. In such circumstances, it was always advisable to store semen in the sperm bank to secure future progeny. It was shocking for all of us as the doctors in Mumbai had never talked about it. In hindsight, I felt they should have, as by not doing so, they were doing a great disservice to their patients. Are cancer patients not expected to procreate? Why did they not think like this? Dr Batia, no doubt, shocked us, but she opened a new door by advising us to store Divyansh's semen in the sperm bank of the hospital. I was not at the hospital then, and these discussions happened in my absence. Sushil discussed the prospect of this with Divyansh, who readily gave his consent to this. By the time I reached the hospital, he was through with the process of storage in the bank. When Divyansh saw me enter his room, he told me, 'Mummy, I have secured my future generation.' I couldn't understand then what he was saying till Sushil narrated the whole story. We are a conservative family where matters concerning sexuality were never discussed openly and never with Divyansh. Divyansh broke this barrier for the first time with me. Initially, I was hesitant to even react but finally did with a gentle smile. My heart thanked Dr Batia profusely that day.

The general environment of the hospital was pleasant. A mall attached to the hospital often saw patients there, even along with their IV line stands. There was a big garden on the other side of the hospital for patients and their caregivers to unwind. But above all, the hospital housed a synagogue where there was a regular prayer congregation. Though we didn't know their religious practices, Sushil and I often went to the synagogue in our solitude to pray for good health for our son. All the nursing staff, doctors and even non-nursing staff served their patients as if they were working to uphold the dignity of human beings. Jews, as I said, are very religious people for whom service to humankind has to be godly. I got to first experience that when we stayed in the hospital. Even the tiniest of work related to patients was done with great alacrity and smiles on their faces. The best part of all this was Divyansh was happy in the facility. I wanted to probe him more. While he was on ablation chemo, I asked him, 'Divyansh, what difference do you find between the experience of taking treatment in Mumbai and over here?' Divyansh took a long pause, turned his face to his right to look at a beautiful hillock through the window, finally turned his face to me, looked into my eyes and whispered, 'Mummy, in Mumbai, I used to feel I was diseased, but here in Jerusalem, I feel I have a disease.' His expression spoke volumes. The Holy Land had begun to have its influence on him. He gradually developed a spiritual wisdom to treat his disease as a mere physical problem, it having made no dent on his mind and soul.

The ablation chemo was a painful process for anyone to undergo. Divyansh was no exception. But what was exceptional about him was a new height of human endurance he had touched by dint of the right connection between his mind and soul, wherein the painful process seemed to just caress him as he moved on. For me, it was a huge relief as I was mentally ready to see the worst as the nursing staff had forewarned us. There were lots of volunteers employed by the hospital whose job was to engage the patients according to their areas of interest. Music, especially playing the guitar, was Divyansh's second passion. One such volunteer was a lady guitarist Ella, who must have been in her forties then. Actually, Ella played a lot of instruments, but for Divyansh, she chose to play the guitar. She would come thrice a week and spend an hour with him. The way Divyansh played the guitar with her always reminded me of his thought that *he had a disease*. Thus, Ella introduced music in his treatment. His age-old nemesis appeared dwarfed by the way he continued to carry on in a new set-up. Then, there were young students' volunteer groups, all mostly in their teens, who came and talked to Divyansh and they generally tried to foster some camaraderie with him. There were times when they sang songs in chorus. One of them, whose name I forget, came always to see Divyansh and talk for hours. All my life, especially with Divyansh, I had never seen medical treatment happening in such a congenial atmosphere, where the anatomy of the body of patients was handled by the doctors and nursing staff, and their minds and souls by angels like such volunteers.

We were fast approaching 9 June, the day chosen for transfer of the donor's cells in Divyansh's body system. As we inched close to the date, all his vital blood parameters were going down, low enough to catch any infection. So he had to be protected from visitors. We, as caregivers, had to keep ourselves fit and healthy so that we could be by his side all the time, even though his vital blood counts were zero due to the ablation chemo. Sushil practised yoga and pranayama, and I generally kept myself engaged around Divyansh and Ananya. I knew it was going to be a new birth of my son, the credit for which had to go to that donor who gave away his body cells for my son. We didn't know him. We would never know him. There was a secrecy clause which restricted disclosure of their names to the patients or their parents up till three years from the date of transplantation.

On 9 June, which was a Tuesday, I woke up early in the morning and said my prayers to the Gods I always worshipped. Sushil, after doing his yoga, did the Buddhist chanting of 'Nam Myoho Renge Kyo'. Dr Or arrived at 10 a.m. with a bag containing the donor's stem cells. The two small pouches were big enough to transfuse a new life to a person like Divyansh. As these pouches were connected to him via IV lines, my eyes were glued to them as if it was not only Divyansh, but I, too, was being transfused with a new life-force. I watched as each drop entered my son's body bit by bit. I felt as if the music of my life was being played before me. Music, which was beautiful as it played, and yet made no sound. In a couple of hours, by noon, the donor's cells were transfused into my son without any issues. I was worried about any unexpected episodes during the process of transplantation, which I had heard happened in some cases. It was a huge relief to us. By evening, Divyansh woke up. As we saw a sense of solace in each other's faces, my hand caressed his cheek and I gave him a flying kiss. The mother in me could read all that his eyes evoked. Maybe he was trying to gauge from me how he had performed in a bigger examination in his life that day, having missed his college examination earlier in the year. My flying kiss, which I had never given in the past, said it all.

Sushil and I went to the hospital synagogue in the evening and sat there for long. We worshipped their Messiah in our own ways and prayed for the full recovery of Divyansh. That night, I stayed with Divyansh. Even though I was woken up every now and then because of frequent nurse visits, the little sleep I got was worth millions. It was a sleep loaded with solace, comfort and hope. I silently thanked the unknown donor who chose to donate his stem cells voluntarily for the cause of my son. I wanted to thank him personally but there was no way I could reach out to him. Later, a realization dawned on me that the best way to thank the donor would be to register myself as a potential donor for needy patients. On our return to Mumbai, taking cue from this thought, Sushil and I got ourselves tested for our blood types and registered as donors for whenever the need arose.

The nurses of the ward felt particularly interested in taking care of Divyansh. Of all the nurses, however, David was the closest to him. He spent his leisure time with Divyansh and they discussed issues of common interest. And their areas of interest matched a lot. When Divyansh was admitted in the Hadassah Hospital, David was due to retire in seven to eight months. I was amazed to see their camaraderie despite a huge age difference. David was such a jovial person that he often danced to the music Divyansh played on his bluetooth speaker in his room. David called him Div and would enter his room in his characteristic style saying, 'Hi, bud!' and Divyansh would respond with a gentle smile. I was happy to see that Divyansh had found a new friend in David and was generally in high spirits in his company. Sushil has written a reminiscence on their vibrant relationship, which can be found towards the end of the book.

After the transfusion of donor cells, it takes about two weeks for their engraftment in the patient's body. Optimally, the blood counts should start in two to three weeks from the date of transplantation. Gaining blood counts meant successful engraftment of the donor's cells. Every day I wondered if Divyansh's blood counts would at all start showing up, and if not, then what? Such unusual thoughts disconcerted me with unknown apprehension, though the doctors and the nurses always appeared confident about it. Till Divyansh's blood counts returned to normal, he had to be protected from all possible sources of infection. The standard blood counts test, CBC, was done daily. To our amazement and also the doctors', Divyansh's blood counts started moving up from the fourteenth day of the transplantation. On the fifteenth day, they shot up more, and the progress continued with every passing day. It was a huge relief for all of us, as it meant the successful engraftment of the donor's cells. We rejoiced at Divyansh's new birth. As a matter of fact, the date of transplantation is taken as day zero in the scheme of treatment protocol. In Divyansh's case, it was 9 June, and then they counted days forward from this date as +1 day, +2 days and so on. This was also the beginning of a new life-cycle and, hence, a rebirth. Divyansh finally achieved his normal blood counts by +21 day, and he was set to be discharged. The doctors were happy with his progress and even remarked that he had shown textbook-style progress. They were particularly appreciative of his determination with which he carried on thus far. Some of them even remarked that Divyansh seldom showed signs of physical pain and the feeling of dejection in the face of the tedious transplantation process, which was rare. The discomfort caused by pain could not match the level of spirit he had raised, and that was why every single time, he was able to channelize the fuel of his pain to the path of recovery.

What now remained was Phase IV of the procedure, which was to be followed up in the day-care facility of the hospital and for which hospitalization was not necessary. We were quite enraptured on the day of discharge. Divyansh was still weak. The nurses were used to seeing him in hospital gowns. When they saw him in blue denims and a T-shirt, they squealed at how different he looked then. One of them brought a wheelchair to take him to the taxi since almost all patients used it as they became very weak after the transplantation. Divyansh politely refused to use the wheelchair and instead preferred walking through the hospital corridors to the taxi. And why not? He always challenged his inner strength every time he faced demanding situations and took it to a different level. That day was no exception. His physical body was undoubtedly weak, but his spirit had become even stronger.

By the time Divyansh was discharged from the hospital, Mridul flew in from Dubai, where he still works, and joined us for a month. That was a big relief for us as Divyansh was very close to him. Anshoo gave him company for a month before the transplantation, and now Mridul would be with him for at least a month after transplantation. Time has taught me that in difficult times, only parents are not sufficient when their children, especially if they are young adults, face challenging situations like this. Anshoo and Mridul were such shining motes who filled this gap and enlivened Divyansh more with their refreshing company. By this time, we were already in the first week of July and were concerned about the reopening of Ananya's school after summer vacations. Considering her need, Sushil advised me to go back to Mumbai with her so that she could join her classes. It was also felt that in a couple of months, Divyansh would expectedly leave Jerusalem after completion of his treatment. Since Mridul had come, Sushil also decided to travel with me, only to come back within a week to join Divyansh for the remaining treatment process. He had been away from his office for more than three months and there were certain pressing matters which he had to attend to. Mridul encouraged us to go, assuring us that he would take care of Divyansh till Sushil rejoined them after a week. It was very difficult for me to leave Divyansh when he perhaps required my unstinting care. I was at the crossroad where, on the one hand, I had to attend to the educational needs of my daughter and on the other hand, my son required my care in his most difficult times. But considering everything, I came back to Mumbai with Ananya and Sushil with a heavy heart. Sushil, of course, went back to join him within a week. As a mother, in hindsight, I realized remorsefully that I shouldn't have left Divyansh then and come back to Mumbai for Ananya's schooling. It flushed me with a terrible feeling. Actually, I realized my horrendous mistake just after reaching Mumbai.

5

MEETING HIS LOST FRIEND

The past is beautiful because one never realizes an emotion at that time. It expands later and thus we don't have complete emotions about the present, only about the past.

—Virginia Woolf

As I write today, I have come to realize how profound this thought is. As I've said earlier, life gives us opportunities for redemption. I also got mine for a mistake, which I will discuss in another chapter.

Divyansh, along with Sushil and Mridul, periodically visited the hospital for follow-up and GvHD. His progress was steady and smooth so far. Gradually, Dr Or began to reduce the doses of various medicines, a welcome sign of Divyansh's physical parameters returning to normalcy.

14 July 2015. It was my birthday and Divyansh was not with me for the first time ever. I was never fond of celebrating my birthday. My kids, Divyansh and Ananya, gave it a new meaning for me when they came into my life. On this birthday, away from Divyansh, I wanted to reflect on his absence. Before I could do anything about it, I received a WhatsApp message. It was a letter from Divyansh in which he not only reflected about himself but also ensured my reflection on my behalf. It emphatically validated that reflections of a mother and son can't stand in isolation. They needed to be done in tandem for their completeness. An excerpt

from the letter is as follows:

> You might not feel like that darling, but then, I have explained that part in my latest poem for you, some people are so special that they are tested that little bit extra and they always manage to move on, even if it involves getting hurt sometimes. *You* are that one person. This is something I strive to learn from you.
>
> No amount of words and gifts can take away the fact that I am not there physically to be with you on your birthday, clap for you while you cut your cake, sing to you, hug you and basically celebrate with you. It does feel very heavy inside when I think of this, but I guess, like I mentioned before, we are special people, Mummy, who are given that extraordinary ability to face whatever test God throws our way with all strength, courage and happily.
>
> Yes I do miss you a lot, Mummy. When my sleep breaks in the night, and my legs start aching, I only wail mentally, 'Mummy!'; when I eat food, Papa's cooking only reminds me of you; when Papa massages my back and front with lotion, I miss your tender touch and, mostly, I just miss you a lot. When you are around, I don't know why but there is something mystical about your motherhood that makes me feel like a child all over again, running into the warm lap of his mother.
>
> Happy birthday, Mummy.

The letter moved me to tears. The feeling of not being with him became more intense. It was annoying. The feeling of helplessness became rather afflicting. Of course, I did cut a cake that day, but all along, my first three fingers holding the knife were gasping for the gentle touch of Divyansh's fingers over them as I moved them to cut the cake.

Towards the end of July, Mridul had to return to work in Dubai as his leave was coming to an end and there was no chance of an extension. It was decided that Sushil would continue alone after his departure for as long as he could go on. As luck would have it, right on the day Mridul was to leave for Dubai by the late night flight, Divyansh had to be admitted to the hospital for CMV infection, the standard treatment of which was anti-viral medicine administered intravenously. It required his hospitalization for at least two weeks. Managing the apartment and kitchen and looking after Divyansh at the same time in the hospital looked too difficult for Sushil to manage alone. He perhaps wished for Mridul to stay back. But considering his job predicament, he advised him to go. More than Sushil, it was going to be a big emotional loss for Divyansh to manage in his absence, more so when he was to be hospitalized again and I was not around. I am sure it must have been equally difficult for Mridul to leave them alone when he was very needed then. It is said: 'I am not going to stop when I am exhausted. I only stop when I am done... Things are never done. That means I will never stop.'

Sushil managed well in Mridul's absence, though it was too taxing for him. Every morning after giving Divyansh his breakfast, he left him alone for a couple of hours in the care of nurses and went back to the apartment to cook food for the day, wash the used utensils and do a little bit of housekeeping. He then came back to the hospital with cooked lunch and dinner, only to return the next morning to go through the same drill. Although the hospital provided food for the patients, it was not for Divyansh's palate due to the difference in food habits of the people of Israel. To overcome the emotional void in Mridul's absence, Divyansh resumed his studies in the hospital itself for the Class 12 board examination next year. It was amazing for the nurses and the doctors who entered his room to see him solving Physics problems with his hand connected to the pouch with the IV line. Come what may, the show must go on. That's what he had practised all his life and that's what he did then. He was inspirational not only for the nurses and doctors but also for the other patients in the ward to whom the nurses would often talk about Divyansh and his never-say-die spirit. I was quite depressed for Divyansh for having missed his Class 12 exams due to his relapse early this year. When he sent me his selfie studying in the hospital, my sagging hopes were rejuvenated. As always, he lent me his helping hand to carry on with my hope. If it doesn't happen today, it shall surely happen tomorrow. I wondered that at his age, boys usually carried bags of books and notebooks to school or college, but Divyansh was carrying two bags: one, of course, of books and the other heavy one full of medicines and related stuff. To my amazement, he struck the right balance between these two bags and moved on with his life, and at the same time, showed us the way to move along.

My youngest sister Shivangi took leave from her office to be with them and joined them after a week. After she went there, I was relieved that she would share the household burden with Sushil and would be excellent company for Divyansh as he gelled well with her. Divyansh was finally discharged from the hospital in the second week of August. After discussion with Dr Or, their return to Mumbai was decided for 9 September, as Divyansh now only required his follow-up, which was possible with a known doctor in Mumbai, Dr Tapan Saikia, in collaboration with Dr Or. It was difficult for me to hold the feeling of exhilaration at my family uniting again, and the day was coming soon.

Divyansh was to return after a new birth. Maybe he himself felt his new birth. He had once written that he was an introvert from the outside and an extrovert from the inside. He must have been talking to himself a lot after he supposedly shed all his medical problems after transplantation. All this led him to broadcast his feeling on a broader canvas of life. There came another poem by him, titled 'Rebirth', which he wrote on 19 August. The poem reflected his thoughts on his doomsday, and how he carried himself amidst all this with the right spirit at his command, acknowledging all those persons who helped him as he moved on. Here is an excerpt:

> Now, as I stand at the precipice of this path,
> I truly understand,
> The true nature of transience, as it always is.
>
> What goes down always comes up,
> The sun always rises after setting,
> What breaks is always rebuilt,
> Sufferings are like weak relations,
> That are broken by the Iron Hand of Time.
> Are some of the lessons,
> This Angelic Cradle taught me.
>
> With an additional layer of perspective,
> My boots shine with new energy,
> As I continue my sojourn,
> Towards eternal heartiness and peace,
> On this path, long, but not bemused.

Actually, it was not only a rebirth for Divyansh but for all of us. Life is not always what we want to have. More often than not, it poses its own challenges. Sometimes the challenges are so harsh that they completely change the path we want to walk on. It is up to us how we face them and take us forward. The tough path we are subjected to tread on, many a time, becomes a path of redemption where a new reality in one's own self is realized. That is rebirth. In fact, we take a lot of rebirths in a single life-cycle before we actually die. This poem and the life experiences of Divyansh culminating into his writing of the poem gave me the wisdom to look at my own life and the obstacles coming my way differently.

Before returning to Mumbai, Sushil took Divyansh to the nearby Malkha Mall for shopping. In the past years, Divyansh had put on a lot of weight due to the side effects of continuous intake of steroids. Steroids, though life-saving drugs, have their own pitfalls. They suppress immunity and make one puffy. Due to prolonged exposure to them, he became too obese to even find the right sized T-shirts in the store. Sushil often told me how Divyansh used to grapple to find his size in apparel and how his exasperation over the process became palpable on his face. After all, he was only in his teens. And he would heave a big sigh of relief when he finally found one. More than Divyansh, it was too much for Sushil to see all this. I realized for the first time how difficult it was to find XXL size and how relieving it was to finally find one for him. It's okay to not be okay, as long as you do not give up. The XXL size could be relieving and enticing: I never knew this paradox. Divyansh, all through the process of finding the right size, was more disturbed at the long wait for his father at the store. That was the reason Sushil never took me along when he went clothes-shopping for Divyansh. He probably wanted to shield two people from the pain: me and Divyansh. I never saw pleasure on their faces when they returned after shopping. I knew what was happening but avoided discussing it. In his wardrobe, though Divyansh had a lot of clothes, sadly, only a few fit him, and so, he would wear those few T-shirts all the time, since the others had become victims of steroids. I often felt irritated when I saw Divyansh wearing the same set of clothes all the time. I regret having done so then.

After the transplantation, Divyansh got his right physique. His weight reduced by at least 30 kg. Sushil wanted to let Divyansh splurge in a fashion store where he could select any clothes without the bother of finding the right size. Let him redeem what he had wished but couldn't get earlier. It was an absolute pleasure for Divyansh as well when he told Sushil with utmost excitement in a Mango store, 'Papa, now, my size is a medium.' On hearing this, Sushil's eyes became moist. He became too numb to react. The happiness and sense of contentment he found in those few words of Divyansh's were worth millions. Words fall short to portray how relieving Divyansh's journey from XXL to M was. After he returned to Mumbai, while I cleaned out all his XXL clothes from his wardrobe, Divyansh held my hand when I removed the last of the lot, an orange T-shirt and said, 'Mummy, don't throw this one. This is the one I wore the maximum number of times and which saved me from embarrassment many times.'

28 August 2015, Rakshabandhan Day. Divyansh was not with his sister, Ananya. As siblings, both were very close to each other. Though the age gap between them was about five-and-a-half years, Divyansh was like a father figure for her in recent years. Ananya was a shy girl and generally kept everything to herself. Pain or pleasure, she didn't normally share with us. That's how she was and we had accepted it. The first word she picked up in her early childhood after Mummy and Papa was Ayya, which was what she called Divyansh, instead of Bhaiya. Over time, as she grew, she started sharing her feelings with Divyansh and only with him. With the passage of time, Divyansh became Bhaiya from Ayya. On this Rakshabandhan Day, to celebrate his brotherhood for Ananya, he wrote her a poem, 'Ayya', where he talked about their journey from Ayya to Bhaiya and read it to her on the phone. It was the most precious gift a brother could give to his sister on this auspicious day. Here's a part of it:

> We both grew up together,
> Although half a dozen winters apart;
> Laughing and playing, crying and fighting,
> Learning and teaching, sleeping and waking,
> As she twisted her tongue,
> To move from 'Ayya' to 'Bhaiya'.

…

I do believe,
Her feelings are a Treasure Chest,
That has gems and stones,
Locked and hidden from all of us.

Sometimes she does open it for me,
And mostly only to me,
Because I know the code to this box;
The word with which she first,
Called me for.

Nothing can be a better gift of life to a brother than to be blessed with a younger sister. Likewise, no one can be as good a protector and guide to a growing girl as her elder brother is.

6

THE MILKY-WHITE-CLAD ANGELS

Gratitude is the fairest blossom which springs from the soul.

—Henry W. Beecher

The date of their return to Mumbai was fast approaching. Dr Reuven Or invited Sushil and Divyansh for dinner to an open-air restaurant outside the city. It was fascinating to experience a doctor in an alien country inviting his patient and his parent for a family dinner. Not just invited them, but came himself to their apartment to pick them up and drove them to the restaurant. Divyansh characteristically wrote a letter addressed to Dr Or, expressing his gratitude for all that he had done for him. Dr Or's relationship with Divyansh, by that time, had transcended the usual boundary of doctor–patient relationships. Divyansh, after the dinner, first read out the letter to the good doctor and his wife Hani, and then handed it over to him. The letter was poignantly written by a patient, who had seen a holy doctor who not only treated him with all compassion but also prayed for him every Sabbath in a synagogue. Dr Or was so moved by that letter that he told Divyansh that it was the priciest gift ever received by him from his patients in his entire career spanning 40 years. After the dinner, Dr Or first dropped them to the apartment before proceeding to his home.

Divyansh decided to do two more things before leaving Jerusalem. First, he wrote a letter addressed to all the nurses of the ward, acknowledging their godly services for his recovery. These nurses were not used to such expression by their patients when they were discharged. Divyansh and Sushil, with prior information, requested them to assemble in their retiring room in the ward and then cut a cake in celebration of their services. Divyansh then read out the letter to all of them. Yevgeni, the chief nurse of the hospital, videographed the proceedings and circulated it not just to many people but also uploaded it on the hospital website. That video became quite a rage in the hospital. This is what Divyansh wrote for them:

Hope is a good thing. Maybe the best of things. And no good thing ever dies.

— Andy Dufresne, *The Shawshank Redemption*

This is exactly what I found here, when I came here after my second relapse of leukaemia. My despair had become outshined by the strongest thing of all, hope. Hope that you all have given me.

What a long journey it has been! But so smooth was the journey that it never felt long. All thanks to you nurses. A patient wants only two things to be fulfilled. Firstly, that he/she is not treated like a patient, but like a normal human being. And secondly, an atmosphere that keeps him/her upbeat all the time. The tough time of the treatment, well, that is taken care of if these two things are provided. You guys not only ensure these with your true 'hospitality' (pun intended) but also work towards ensuring this in such a natural manner that it never looks pretentious. Always having that ever-shining glow on your faces, coupled with beautiful smiles, an energetic attitude and most importantly, the calmness with which you handle even the most critical of situations are just the right things that a patient and his/her attendant need when they come to your ward, trembling with apprehension and uncertainty. Your absolute dedication and ever-encouraging support for the patient makes (at least it made me) one feel, 'Yes, everything will be taken care of by them. No need to worry.'

Thank you, Yevgeni, Bella, David, Neta, Marina, Alisa, Nasrine, Ami, Veronica, Chana Apter, Chana Ephrat, Chana Budin, Shoshi, Ayelet (thanks for teaching me perspective drawing), Ella (for bringing music into my treatment), Rut, Essa, Naomi, Zachary, Avital, Orit, Ilana, Elisheva, Edvard, Shira, Rinat, Chana Spiro, Tzuf, Maria, Esther, Helena, Alexander (I will learn and speak Hebrew the next time we meet), Carmel, Ori (I like your hairstyle!), Yochi, Hadass, Ahmed Sheber, Ahmed Abu Diab, Limor, Shadah, Michal and Chava (you were the first one to take my blood for the tests). And also, thank you Aden and the few other volunteers who have taken up health care service for national duty. You are, indeed, truly serving your nation, and more, importantly, humanity. This was, indeed, 'the best day of my life'.

Always Grateful,

6 September 2015   Divyansh Atman

The letter moved some of the nurses to tears. It seemed it was not only the *best day of life* for Divyansh, but perhaps, also for them.

Next up, a day after, he wrote another letter addressed to all the doctors of the ward and read it out to them in their conference hall before handing it over to them. The doctors were full of appreciation for Divyansh and even commented that this was rare where a patient was giving more than the fees. Here goes Divyansh's letter for them:

Health is wealth.

And only its absence makes you realize its true value. One may have all the talents, wealth, opportunities, but infirmity is something that nullifies them all.

Dear doctors, it may be your daily job to see patients, attend to their complaints and plan the line of treatment to be followed. Being in the BMT department, it may be commonplace for you to perform BMTs frequently. The bag that carries the bone marrow stem cells may seem like any other haemoglobin bag. You may feel that you are just 'doing your job'. Let me tell you how I see this as a patient.

The bag containing the stem cells is the life that you doctors have given me after painstakingly monitoring, searching and finding it suitable to be transplanted into me. You have given me a new life, a life that has taken birth from the ashes of an old life of unending chemotherapy, torturous side effects and often painful injections—a life filled with despair and uncertainty. Now, because of you, I can breathe a new life, live it to the fullest and accomplish my dreams. The same clothes that I would stretch and squeeze to fit into now droop from my body. I feel lighter and better. The same mind that worked at only half its efficiency now is always eager to work at its fullest. Cancer is the emperor of all maladies. You have crushed this emperor with all your might and saved me from its tyranny. This is what you do so 'frequently', the regular job you do daily.

Thank you, Dr Reuven Or, Dr Michael Shapira, Dr Alex, Dr Sigal, Dr Avni, Dr Vipul (lucky to find a doctor from my country here!) and all other doctors who did their 'daily job' for me. May God really bless you. And please convey my thanks to Dr Mehrovich, the radiologist.

Yours gratefully,
6 September 2015   Divyansh Atman

Divyansh was all set to leave Israel with a rechristened soul, endowed with the spirit of the holy land of Jerusalem.

On 9 September 2015, as they were about to leave the apartment, Divyansh took his selfie in a new avatar, all in medium-sized clothes and sent it to me with a caption: 'COMING BACK'.

One doesn't go to Jerusalem, one returns to it.
That's one of its mysteries.

7

STRONGER THAN EVER BEFORE

Divyansh was completely engrossed in writing a poem. I was curious to know what he was writing. Since his return from Jerusalem, he had completely switched himself onto study mode to prepare for the Class 12 board examination and other engineering entrance tests. He was still very weak and, so, his carrying on with an intense load of studies often made me nervous. It gave me a reprieve when I saw him writing a poem that must have been a welcome break for him too from routine and rote studies. He seemed to have completely left behind his turbulent past and moved on with a revitalized spirit after his transplantation. A few days before this, he had texted me a message which summed his new-found outlook: 'Today I found a Decmax tablet lying completely crushed and powdered in my wallet. So symbolic.'

Decmax was a steroid which he was exposed to for a long time, and which I talked about earlier.

After dinner, I curiously asked him, 'Divyansh, I think you were writing a poem. If you have finished, can you tell me about it?'

'Mummy, I have just finished writing a poem titled "Blaze". Couple of days back, Ms Wadia requested me to write a poem on one of the five elements of life, and to recite it in a poetry festival on this theme, under the aegis of 100 Thousand Poets for Change at Mumbai Kitab Khana on 18 October. I have chosen to write on fire,' Divyansh replied.

100 Thousand Poets for Change (100TPC) is a global movement inviting poets from across the world to join them to celebrate peace and sustainability through poetry. The poems read by the poets are compiled in a book form and sent to the archives of the Stanford University. When Ms Wadia had read some of Divyansh's poems earlier, she was quite impressed by the originality of underlying thoughts and his writing skills. Her appetite to read more by him grew. And why not? Divyansh had been her blue-eyed student. She wanted him to showcase his talent on a bigger platform like 100TPC. This was the first occasion when Divyansh's work would get some publicity and of course, its publication for archiving in one of the top universities of the world. So, on 18 October, Divyansh, clad in a green cap and brown-and-white striped polo T-shirt, went to Kitab Khana along with Sushil. When his turn came, he went to the dais and confidently recited 'Blaze', his own inner fire very thoughtfully portrayed through this poem. As he was reading it, Ms Wadia drew herself close to him and gave him an affectionate look. The recitation was followed by thunderous applause from the audience. The poem was finally published in a book titled *I Believe* and was sent to Stanford University for archiving. This was the first time that Divyansh's literary skill reached a wider public domain and was recognized. The holy spirit of Jerusalem seemed to have ignited him, and that's why he talked about fire in metaphysical form, which we must rekindle in ourselves to keep our spirit high. He wrote in the concluding part of the poem:

Nerves of steel,
A rock-strong resilience,
Burning determination,
Radiant visage,
Are all the various traits,
Carefully tested by this Master,
Who can burn those who give up,

And strengthen those who don't.
Look into the fire, my friends,

Look at its profoundness,
And rekindle the fire in you,
To make the spirit strong,
Stronger than ever before.

Over a period of time, along with studying for the exams, Divyansh explored himself more and more in writing poetry. What amazed me about his writing was his originality of ideas and the way they were conveyed through the well-knit ensemble of words where each word would convey the undertone of the thought he wanted to convey.

Diwali was round the corner. This was the first Diwali after four years that we were all planning to celebrate with great gusto. I was busy preparing our home for the occasion. While I made rangolis at the entrance of the main door, Divyansh was absorbed in making a rangoli of words on his literary canvas. Yes, he was busy writing a poem on Diwali. I wondered what he would write on Diwali other than the mundane things we normally do. His interpretation and articulation of the celebration of Diwali was on a different paradigm, though. He felt that Diwali, the festival of lights, was considered the triumph of good over evil. Should the celebration of this festival end with lighting candles, sharing sweets and bursting crackers? The real test of the celebration lay in how we unleashed the light of righteousness, knowledge and principles within ourselves and spread warmth all over. The world needed this. The festival of Diwali, thus, should transcend beyond the realm of just being a festival of lights. With this thought in mind, he unleashed his wordplay and beautifully wove this theme in his poem. It read like this:

Today in the Kal-Yug (The Dark Age),
This day is a testament,

That the dark can never conquer the light,
The light of knowledge, the light of righteousness, the
light of principles,
Which is the triumvirate,
That will burn bright, and radiant,
For eternity, and through eternal darkness.

This Diwali, unleash this trinity within you,
And let it burn with omnipotence,
Kindness is the light that will spread,
Goodness is the crackle that will echo,
Happiness is the warmth that will spread,
Inviting all the comfort of contentment,
Enriching all the conscience possessed,
And being fuelled by blessings, from those,
The flame hath touched.

When I read this poem, I took some time to grasp its undertone.
When I was his age, Diwali for me meant celebration, celebration
and only celebration. Divyansh wrote this poem when he was
hardly 18 years old. It was unfathomable for me to discern how
so much wisdom had sprouted in him. Was it battling his nemesis
all through his teens that made him grow intellectually beyond
his age? While I was always proud of him for showing such
exceptional thoughts, I often felt sad that he was showing such
high maturity—why was he not behaving like a person his age
would? I wanted him to enjoy his life, spend time with his (girl)
friends, come home late, where I would rebuke him on coming
late. In a word: normal. While Divyansh was deprived of all this
age-specific fun, I too felt deprived of seeing him have all these
youthful shenanigans and my irritable response to it at times. I
craved for experiences that allowed such irritation and annoyance
between him and me, so that like any normal mother, I could
also scold him. Sadly, he never gave me any room to do all this

with him. Over time, I learnt to live with this affliction.

At his study table, Divyansh always kept two souvenirs gifted by his two revered gurus: a brass image of a dancing Natraj gifted by Raji Madam, his yoga teacher, and a Laughing Buddha from Ms Wadia. The Natraj (Lord Shiva) in the dancing form is considered a symbolic synthesis of the most important aspects of Hinduism. It symbolizes the cosmic cycles of creation and destruction, as well as the daily rhythm of birth and death. The dance represents synthesis of the five principal aspects of eternal energy: creation, destruction, preservation, salvation and illusion. In contrast to this, the Laughing Buddha depicts plenitude of one's wishes for wealth, happiness and satisfaction. The wealth the Laughing Buddha inspired Divyansh to earn was the wealth of knowledge, contentment, gratitude, perseverance and tolerance. In contrast to this, materially, too, in his own sphere, he enjoyed his life with the latest fashion wear, gadgets and he even had all the details of the latest cars the world over, though his father then just owned a small car, a Santro. Remarkably, he knew the right balance between the two nuanced meanings of wealth. Divyansh made conscious endeavours to assimilate the true import of the symbolism represented by the two portraits in his life. He once confessed to me that whenever he looked at the Natraj, he felt a sense of empowerment. Over time, the Laughing Buddha accumulated dust in its small pores which was difficult to clean. Divyansh found beauty and a life lesson even from that dusty Laughing Buddha. One day, he wrote to Ms Wadia:

> Hello Ma'am. Remember the Laughing Buddha you had gifted me when I came to you for classes? The Laughing Buddha, it is said, always comes as a gift. Today, almost three years later, its base polish has chipped off a bit and it has an affinity for dust. But still, his smile is as ebullient as the first time I saw it. Your fifth legacy personified, Ma'am. Being happy under all circumstances.

To me, he manifested true embodiment of the spirit of life philosophy conveyed by these two portraits. I am sure that whatever he was studying for the examination, he consciously tried to lift his learning to this level.

One day, Divyansh, in a thoughtful mood, asked his father, 'What do you think I am: introvert or extrovert?'

'What makes you ask this question?' Sushil asked him return.

'No, nothing specific. I was generally asking your view about me,' Divyansh replied vaguely.

'Look, to me, you are neither introvert nor extrovert. You have a nice blend of both of them in you,' Sushil too said vaguely.

The discussion didn't stop there. He wanted to know more from Sushil but Sushil wasn't forthcoming. The quest of finding the right answer led him to first introspect, then reflect and the result was his next poem 'The Introvert', where, towards the end of the poem, he discovers what he is.

> The Introvert, to an Extrovert,
> Is a stiff, ungenial snob,
> The pillow to prick the thorn,
> The specimen to try pranks on.
> But don't ever be mistaken,
> What shows, is not what is,
> The Introvert is a world in itself,
> A world, unique and profound.
> ...
> Introverts, be proud (be shy),
> You are a shining mote (a dim shadow),
> Unapologetic, uninhibited (apologetic, inhibited),
> And an Extrovert (an Introvert),
> Within (on the outside).
> That's all.

Late in the evening, when Divyansh gave Sushil this poem to read, perhaps he also found the right answer to his question which he couldn't give earlier in the day: introverted from the outside and extroverted from the inside.

Apart from the Class 12 board exams, to prepare for various engineering entrance tests, Divyansh had joined a local coaching centre for this purpose. But after his return from Jerusalem, it was not advisable to attend classroom coaching set-up as he was weak and there was a fear of catching infection. Mr Pravin Tyagi, who was the head of the coaching centre, obliged us by sending his teachers to our home to teach Divyansh and prepare him for the tests. Mr Tyagi was a noble person who felt that sincere students like Divyansh needed to be supported in whatever way possible. Surprisingly, he never charged us an extra penny for this, though Sushil insisted on it. Almost all the teachers who came home to teach Divyansh were fresh IIT graduates who had chosen to join coaching classes instead of serving industries. The age gap between them and Divyansh was not much. The pleasure of a sincere students like Divyansh and being taught by young teachers like them created perfect harmony for teaching. I myself was witness to their synergy where the teacher and the student would crack jokes and laugh together. The teachers often shared with us how much pleasure they felt in teaching him. They were very happy with his utmost sincerity considering the hardships he had to go through. Whenever the teachers came to teach him, I ensured that I served them delectable dishes and generally made sure they were properly taken care of as long as they were at our home. I don't know why, but I felt an inexplicable satisfaction taking care of their palates. I never considered them different from Divyansh, and so, when I served them, it felt like I was serving my son. Initially, they resisted being served food or tea. However, in time, they shed their inhibitions and developed a liking for my food. I would plan in advance whenever a teacher was due to come. Saurav, the teacher who taught him Physics, texted him one day: '*Tumhari mummy ka haath ka khana is heavenly. Never got a chance to tell her this, bol dena unhe*' (Your mother is an excellent cook. Never got a chance to tell her. Please convey my comment to her). More exciting was Divyansh's reply to this message. He texted: 'And I must confess to you, my mummy took special care in preparing something every time you all came.' Divyansh developed a strong bond with them. My desire to serve them food, perhaps, was an implicit attempt to reinforce that bond.

2016 was around the corner. I only wished the new year would herald a new life for Divyansh. But I thought this at the beginning of many past years, and every new year would disappoint us. In the first week of January, Divyansh received a call from Yevgeni, the chief nurse of the BMT department of the Hadassah Hospital, requesting him to send a video of his speech for David's retirement function. Since Divyansh's return from Jerusalem, he was in regular touch with David and his other Israeli friends. He was aware of his upcoming retirement and had thought about what he could do for this occasion. And here came the invitation from Yevgeni. He immediately promised to send him the video as desired in a couple of days. When Sushil came back from work that evening, Divyansh discussed Yevgeni's request with us. Of all the patients David had served, and it must have been in thousands, Sushil wondered why Divyansh was chosen to deliver the valedictory speech. He told Divyansh that it was his honour to have been chosen by Yevgeni to reflect on David at his retirement function. Writing being Divyansh's forte, he wrote a stirring speech and delivered it eloquently and poignantly as Sushil recorded. The video was mailed to Yevgeni. Yevgeni, in return, sent him the video of David's retirement function, where Divyansh's speech was played on a giant screen. We could see all the doctors, nurses and other support staff with whom we were quite familiar now moved to tears as his speech progressed. David couldn't believe his eyes at what he was witnessing then. Not just him but all those present there exuded the utmost admiration for Divyansh. The applause after the speech was as much for David's distinguished services to the hospital as they were for Divyansh in the way he understood and articulated about David. Long live, David, you are a wonderful person who Divyansh always kept close to his heart.

27 January 2016, Divyansh's nineteenth birthday. We had many plans to make that a big day. Divyansh too was very happy. He characteristically believed in meaningful celebration of days like this. Likewise, he always made sure our birthdays and wedding anniversary were celebrated blissfully. On such occasions, his biggest gift to us had been his letters, which he would give us after the celebration. Those letters are precious gems. When he wrote about me, it sometimes felt like he knew me more than even I did myself. We took him to his favourite eating joint Punjab Grill at the famous Palladium Mall in Mumbai. After the dinner, Sushil casually asked him to reflect on his past years. Divyansh very thoughtfully said, 'Today, I complete my teenage days. My entire teenage life went in ceaseless struggle. But I don't harbour any grudge about it. I have moved on in my life and hope to keep moving like this.' Sushil got emotional listening to his feelings, and said, 'I agree, Divyansh. You may have missed the tantalizing taste of your teenaged life, but in return, you have been compensated with supreme wisdom which time has bestowed upon you, and of which we too are beneficiaries.' When Sushil drove us back home, I looked across the window to the distant Haji Ali Dargah, reminiscing about Divyansh's turbulent teenaged days.

Like us, Mridul too waited for Divyansh's birthday. He would make sure to send him personal notes and gifts of Divyansh's liking. This birthday was no different. He texted his birthday wishes for Divyansh. His vivid description about Divyansh was so real that I have to share that here.

Such a year this has been! Your first year into adulthood … and it's beautifully coincidental how it has also been your first year into the beginning of a new chapter in your life post the treatment. And as you enter the last year of your teens, I wonder and I am compelled to tell you how graciously you have handled your teens. Apparently, these are known to be the years when majority of the lot goes awry.

But not you! You have been the best and a very un-teenager-like teenager. So composed. So mature. No troubles at all for the parents and guardians. Following what should be followed to the T.

The only thing which I felt needed a slight change was your holding back yourself, the slight losing of your fun side which would rear into the world unabashedly … and I had hinted this on your last birthday.

And today after a year, I can proudly say that you have definitely moved towards becoming the naughtier, funnier version of yourself … the way you used to be as a kid. I don't know if you have worked towards it knowingly or subconsciously, but whatever it is that inspires you or however it is that you are able to do it, you must keep doing it. I think this is the biggest gift that adulthood has given you. I love to see this new version of you who goes out no-holds-barred to be a little more naughty and a little less serious.

And I wish for you on this birthday, that you keep doing this all your life, being the kid that you used to be … laughing and having fun and pulling pranks and being creative all your way through this game called life… You are playing it with panache… Happy 19th birthday, dearest Divyansh!

Yes, Divyansh did reply to Mridul. He wrote:

Dear Bhaiya,

First of all, thanks for the good wishes. Probably one of the reasons why I would hold back and keep to myself earlier was maybe because I was never truly happy from inside and never really felt really good, no matter how much I tried. My entire teenage life had been unfortunately struck by something unfortunate, which I spent these years battling, along with other things.

Last year, just around this time, I was down with a very bad headache and fever. I remember, I cried at least 10 times on my birthday. And you know what happened subsequently… My treatment, and ultimate triumph, is one of the biggest gifts I could take from this year. And you being there in the time of my transformation was the biggest gift you could have given me. So you don't need to worry about the cap!

As you said about me going back to being what I was in my childhood, I would say that yes, this entire journey has transformed my personality immensely, physically, mentally and spiritually. I have become more expressive. I have been able to imbibe all that was missing from my personality, in my journey of Jerusalem. So I guess, that's what it is! A new immunity and a more equipped, and amiable personality! (Divyansh)

After reading the thoughts they shared with each other, I felt the completeness of Divyansh's birthday celebration.

8

NERVES OF STEEL

For a few days before his birthday, Divyansh had been experiencing excruciating pain in his left leg. Sushil discussed it with Dr Or on the phone, and he prescribed some medicine to give him relief. However, the pain kept coming back. Dr Tapan Saikia alerted us to something potentially sinister and advised his CSF and bone marrow tests as well. Since Divyansh's board examination were at hand, Dr Saikia advised us to do this after it was over. Divyansh patiently managed his studies with intermittent pain. But any pain that Divyansh went through had me shuddering from past recollections.

Sushil's mother, Divyansh's grandmother (dadi), had not been keeping well since the past few months. She had almost become bed-ridden and, after our return from Jerusalem, Sushil and I often visited Patna to see her. I really wanted to spend time with her but Divyansh too needed my constant attention since Jerusalem. Despite my strong desire to be by her side for a few days, I couldn't. I ended up making occasional short visits, and that too because Divyansh coaxed me to go to Patna with Sushil to see his grandmother. Over a period of time, he had won my confidence regarding Ananya's care, which he did very well in my absence. It was painful for Sushil, too, to divide his attention thus. They were five brothers and one sister in Sushil's big joint family, where all four of his older brothers, their wives and children stayed under one roof under the guiding care of his father. Sushil's father, Dr Kedar Nath Poddar, was an authority in law in Bihar, was a professor in Patna Law College and later became the principal of this college before his retirement. He was quite an active person socially and was hugely popular amongst the students he had taught and the teaching fraternity in general. His personality was so majestic that his mere presence at home in Patna invigorated it with warmth and freshness. Someone had commented that Divyansh was a true replica of his grandfather. His gentle smile reminded me of his grandfather. Keeping the family structure in mind, Sushil had some solace that his mother was being properly taken care of in his absence at Patna. But at the end of the day, his mother had five sons and a daughter, of whom four sons were always there to take care of her, but for Sushil, she was the only mother who he craved to serve and take care of when she actually needed it. Sushil still harbours guilt about not attending to her physically in the manner he wanted to. But that's how our lives had been. For the past seven years, we had been constantly living on the edge and still trying to discharge all the responsibilities of our own family, extended family and social ones. Sushil has a terrific sense of managing all his responsibilities despite difficulties in plenty. All this, besides his own official responsibilities. He is sincere to the core. Once Divyansh had written to him:

Papa,

Sometimes I really feel for you. I don't know how you manage to stand up against all odds every time. And it is not even like you have any one to fall back on. We are just a meagre portion of your refuge. The manner in which you had to ultimately go and get involved ... well, that is fate. But you don't worry, Papa. Let me grow up and stand on my feet. Then I promise, you will always have my support and will not have to worry about anything. You will live with all

peace and tranquillity. That is my promise to you. All you
need to do is wait.

Whatever came his way, Sushil took it in his stride, tried to do
his best to move forward and led us from the front.

On 7 February 2016, Sushil got a call from his eldest
brother Shankar, Mridul and Anshoo's father, about the death
of his mother in the morning. Divyansh's exams had just begun.
Besides, he was still getting pain attacks in his legs and, therefore,
required care from at least one of us. I talked to Divyansh about
his readiness to manage himself and Ananya alone till we came
back from Patna. He not only advised me to go with Sushil but
also gave Sushil a letter for his grandmother to read out to her
before she was cremated. I could see his strong urge to make it
to her funeral, but in the face of his on going exams, he couldn't.
Except for his childhood days, he had hardly spent any significant
time with his grandparents as he was battling his own problems
for the last seven years. The craving to meet them had always
run deep in him, though it was hardly perceptible to us. He
was mindful of missing an important chapter of his life with
them that his other cousins got. Sometimes, the truth is deeper
than experience. It is beyond our discernment. The truth of the
deep love and affection which Divyansh had for his grandparents,
perhaps we never knew fully. And the only way to know his truth
is to share it as I write his story. The only experience I had was
to see him sad for not being able to make it.

We went to Patna to attend her last rites. Sushil read out
Divyansh's letter to his grandmother before her cremation. He
wrote:

Dear Dadiji,

I shall ever be in deep sorrow for not having been able to
meet you. My condition was such that despite my strong
desire to see you, I couldn't. Now, as I reminisce the time

spent with you, I become very emotional. Alas, were I able to meet you! Please treat the presence of Papa and Mummy as mine too. I will pray to the Gods for your eternal peace. You will always remain in my memory.

Divyansh

When I read his letter, it only drenched me with the regret of not attending the last rites of my beloved mother-in-law with my children. I could only shed extra tears for Divyansh and Ananya as well.

When we went back to Patna after a few days for her shraddh ceremony, I saw a message thread between Divyansh and Sushil on the mobile phone:

Divyansh: In shraddh, you will be shaving your head as well?

Papa: Yes.

Divyansh: Don't shave your moustache but your hair will come back rapidly.

Papa: Looks like. You appear to understand finer nuances of my hair better.

Divyansh: I understand fine nuances of hair in general. Seven years of experience.

The reason I quote this conversation is to highlight how sportingly Divyansh articulated his understanding about the finer nuances of hair based on seven years of experience of losing it, off and on, and managing himself without it.

Divyansh managed to finish his board exams despite intense pain in his legs. I was apprehensive about whether he could even finish them. Divyansh had nerves of steel, a phrase he used for himself in one of his poems. The day he finished his exams, Sushil expressed his exultation by texting him a message:

Dear Divyansh,

24 July 2015. Do you remember this date?

Maybe you do. From this day you had started again preparing for the board exams from the Hadassah Hospital after a long lull, when you had to be re-admitted for CMV infection. It was your own resolve to resume your study from this day and your hospitalization couldn't dent your resolve. You made a beginning with the conviction 'I shall make it this time'. The resolve was quite palpable. I could notice that. I, however, thought this time you can make it. This was the difference between you and me. The difference between 'shall' and 'can'. I thought let's take one step at a time. Will see as the days go by. From thereon, we moved step by step. Your resolve stood rock solid all along. However, I was apprehensive throughout. You always tried to allay my apprehension whenever it became visible to you. Today, as you have completed your exams, notwithstanding very patchy and troublesome days in between, I feel jubilant not only on completion of your exam, but more because of the way you carried yourself in the past few months in this pursuit. Success is not only achieving mundane desired results but also the manner in which it is achieved. To me, the manner stands much, much more important in your case. As for results, it is already out for me. Today, Mummy, Ananya and I, along with you feel triumphant on all that you have done for yourself and for us too, in caring for our sentiments, of redeeming lost ground.

'What lies behind us and what lies before us are nothing compared to what lies within us.'

My belief in this thought has been reinforced.

Bravo Divyansh. God bless.

Early in March, we got a call from Dr Reuven Or about his forthcoming visit to Mumbai with his wife, Hani. A pharmaceutical company had invited him to deliver a talk on BMT. On hearing this, Sushil requested him to visit our home. It was unimaginable to expect Dr Or, who we in general, and Divyansh in particular, revered so much, would come all the way from Israel and visit our home someday. Sushil wanted to make the most of the small window of opportunity coming our way by inviting them to bless our home. Dr Or wholeheartedly accepted our invite. Towards the end of their visit, they came one evening and spent almost three hours with us. I had prepared assorted Indian cuisine for them to savour. I knew from my close interactions with Dr Or in Jerusalem that he was very fond of Indian dishes. They thoroughly relished the food. After the dinner, we discussed the recent episodes of pain in Divyansh's legs. Prima-facie, he didn't apprehend anything major, however, he suggested that we plan a trip to Jerusalem in the next month after Divyansh was done with various entrance tests for his complete follow-up. I saw his benevolent side when I found him interacting with Divyansh, talking about what he had planned for his career and how he could help him in his pursuit. He even tried to advise him to look for his future in Israel where he would help him in every way. The next day we hosted a get-together in a nearby banquet hall in their honour, where Dr Or's other friends, some of who were also known to us, were invited.

Divyansh's preparation for his various forthcoming entrance tests was in full swing. The teachers who came home to teach him were more than satisfied and happy with his preparation. They were particularly appreciative of his level of dedication culminating in his well-preparedness, despite losing almost nine months on account of treatment and the vigour with which he resumed his studies after coming back from Jerusalem. They would often tell us that they quoted him as an example of dedication to so many students. It seemed success was bound to come and the only thing that could keep it away from him was his destiny. He had enshrined the spirit of the Bhagavad Gita in himself after reading it and established his utmost faith in his own karma, unconcerned with the universal grand design of his life which his destiny would choose. The praise his teachers showered on him often transported me to a dream where I saw Divyansh studying in one of the prestigious IITs. Actually, I only dreamt about IIT Mumbai for Computer Engineering, his favourite subject, for the simple reason that I couldn't have sent him away from us as he required our continuous support. Whenever I discussed the prospect of my dream becoming a reality with Divyansh, he only smiled. He wouldn't utter a single word. I have seen very few people like Divyansh, who stood so humble before his success and never envied the success of his friends though there were plenty who envied him. These sore feelings of others flushed me with anguish. I felt deep hurt when I saw this happening with him. Divyansh was earning his success, inch by inch, each day, by dint of his hard labour and by challenging his own physical limits. How could he be compared with anyone or how could someone compare themselves with him? His path to destiny was different, full of obstacles and ceaseless challenges that he overcame alongside his studies. Divyansh repeatedly told me that he always compared himself with himself only. He had set his own benchmark of success, the essence of which lay in utmost devotion to his duties without bothering much about success. He celebrated each day of his unflinching faith in his own karma as success. That was perhaps the reason for his humility about his achievements, because by then, he had celebrated the success of each day of karma culminating into that achievement.

There were three to four examinations lined up for the first fortnight of April. The first one amongst them was the much celebrated JEE (Main). For a week before this exam, the episodes of frequent attacks of leg pains increased, coupled with some mysterious neurological disturbances on his face. The doctors were clueless about it. The only advice they gave was to go through a series of tests. We were ready for it but only after his exams. The strange facial neurological disturbances sometimes made him black out for some time. I knew for sure that he was going through some complications post transplantation. There was nothing much we could have done then but wait for the exams to get over and then travel to Jerusalem for follow-ups. A day before the JEE (Main) examination, his Math teacher Mahaveer Godhra came home to wish him good luck. He said Divyansh was all set to get what he aspired for. But that day, by evening, the episodes of facial disturbances and black outs became more frequent. The kind of irritation and apprehension I felt was not visible in Divyansh's demeanour. He was cool and composed. The next morning, Divyansh woke up in a not-so-good-state and prepared to leave for the examination centre. Sushil accompanied him. Seeing him sleeping in the car on the way petrified Sushil. He expected something to happen. After they had left, I dropped Ananya to school, went to the nearby Babulnath Temple and sat for hours praying for the success of my son. Divyansh would be thoroughly dejected if something were to happen to him on that day. Divyansh had done his karma. I was doing mine at the Babulnath Temple. It was now God's turn to bestow upon my son his blessings. I stayed there and prayed till Sushil called after the exam.

After Divyansh has entered the centre, Sushil waited for him till he came out. Before he could ask him anything, Divyansh painfully told him that he had a mental black out before the exam, which made him attempt hardly a few questions. He was engulfed with heavy sleepiness which he couldn't overcome. Sushil listened to him coolly, patted his shoulder and said, 'Don't worry my dear son; you are destined for bigger success in your life.'

Divyansh had requested Sushil to take him to the Siddhi Vinayak Temple after the exam on the way back home. Though he hadn't done well, he insisted on going to the temple so they went and took God's blessings. Divyansh's piety to God was always quiet but profound.

When they came back and I heard all that had happened with Divyansh during the exam, I was devastated. I again questioned the credibility of the Gods I worshipped. Lord Shiva of the Babulnath Temple seemed to have betrayed Divyansh with his blessings.

Or were his blessings reserved for something else in the coming days?

In the other entrance tests, Divyansh did fairly well. But I was still bemused.

ॐ

9

YOU SEE, I HAVE RENOUNCED FEAR

This time, Anshoo accompanied Sushil and Divyansh when they flew to Jerusalem in the third week of April for a follow-up with Dr Reuven Or. Before their departure, I prayed for their successful trip, but more than that, for reassuring news of Divyansh's well-being after his check-up. The day they reached Jerusalem, it was raining, with strong gusty winds. Navdeep Singh came to their apartment with breakfast for them. Later, he took them to the hospital and remained with them till the evening. At his first look at Divyansh, Dr Or exasperatedly said that he apprehended some major problem. Sushil was shaken to hear that. The first question that came to his mind was, could the transplantation go awry? If yes, what then? Divyansh was at a loss. He was still trying to figure out what had happened to him. Back in Mumbai, I was too worried. I was only waiting for Sushil's call to hear the result of the follow-up. Sushil called me a couple of times during the day but nothing conclusive had been discovered. However, the tone and tenor of his voice was enough to indicate that everything was not alright. I was reflecting on Divyansh's life, full of incessant stumbling blocks, one after the other: they refused to abate. But above all, beyond perhaps even God, I had faith in Divyansh and Dr Or. Whatever happened, Dr Or would handle it and show us the way to move forward.

The CNS and bone marrow tests were done, which turned out to be negative to our huge relief, else it would have just negated the benefit of transplantation altogether. But Dr Or was not content. There was something manifesting through those leg pains and the neurological disturbances on Divyansh's face. A CT scan revealed some serious complications post transplantation, which required immediate intervention. The complications he was diagnosed with by Dr Or were rare and they happened in very few reported cases. When Dr Or told Divyansh about the challenges he was facing and the impending treatment protocol, he patiently listened and asked him when he was done, 'Does this mean that the transplantation has failed in my case?' Dr Or said, 'Not at all, but whatever it is, it requires a thorough treatment and future follow-up.' Hearing this, Sushil told Dr Or that he was ready to do everything for his betterment. Seeing the resolve and well-composed demeanour of Divyansh, Dr Or smilingly told them not to worry. He would try his best to fix the problem. He asked them to come back in three days by which time he would finalize the best treatment option. In the evening, Sushil first broke the relieving news to me about the CNS and bone marrow tests being negative, and then the heart-breaking news of complications in the manner Dr Or perceived. I was more perturbed about what must be going on in Divyansh's mind. Oh, I should have been there with him! How would I face him if something wrong happened? However, the past experiences gave me a reassuring feeling about Divyansh. He always stood calm when any devastating news like this was broken to him. Despite the extremities of the circumstances he was in, I never felt I would lose him. Through his resilient personality, he not only kept himself well poised, but also assiduously ensured that we remained unruffled to face the challenges. Many a time, our friends complimented us on the way we handled Divyansh's challenging situations. They were wrong. It was Divyansh who was guiding us all the way as he moved on while facing problems. I thought it would be very tough for Sushil to manage alone. When I talked to Divyansh, he sounded like nothing had happened to him. Whenever I was deeply anxious, talking to Divyansh unfailingly soothed me and worked therapeutically on me. He made me feel fine but there was some profound thought brewing in his mind which was fuelled by his heroic soul.

22 April 2016. The next day morning, he wrote a poem for himself. The poem was titled 'Catharsis'. The poem was about his conversation with God, the pouring out of his emotion-laden heart—and that was catharsis. Divyansh, in the face of ceaseless adversities in his life, again stood completely bowed before God, acknowledging his supremacy with deference in the backdrop of his grand design, and tried to invoke godliness in himself to take charge of his own life to do his karma. Through this poem, he demonstrated unrelenting faith in his own spirit to rise like a phoenix from ashes every time circumstances were stacked against him. Some excerpts:

> I will have unconditional implicit faith,
> In your Grand design,
> And never blame You, or fate,
> For misfortune that may become mine.

> I will wield my own plough,
> I will cultivate my own land,
> I will do all my karma,
> And embrace whatever comes, with warm, open hands.

> You see, I have renounced fear,
> And over optimism and expectation.
> I will move ahead from here,
> With a numbness tempered by determination,
> guts, patience
> And denial.

> I will be smiling and singing all along,
> And catching the horns of what comes my way,
> With an unrelenting, aggressive battle cry.

The poem shows Divyansh's strong resolve in the face of misfortunes which never ended. It made our resolve even stronger. This poem became quite popular in the course of time and was recited on many occasions, which I will discuss in other chapters. When Divyansh gave the poem to Sushil to read, he felt humbled to read it. The poem evoked courage, fortitude and immense optimism in Divyansh as he moved through hindrances in his life and how much stronger he eventually emerged after each round of such obstacles. Each and every word of the poem owed its origin to the experiences his life had taught him. A part of this indefatigable spirit Divyansh inherited from his father. Sushil is one person who never gave up till he was pushed to the wall. Even then, he would try ways to move forward. Despite so many problems with Divyansh, he unfailingly stood rock solid with his calm persona and relentlessly explored all possible avenues of treatment. Even now, when Dr Or told him about Divyansh's latest medical complication, he didn't give up and went along with Dr Or to try other treatment options. But, unlike Divyansh, he never had the opportunity for catharsis. He would absorb whatever came his way and move on with a smile on his face. In a way, Divyansh and Sushil fully complemented each other, and that's why they together became the epitome of father–son relationship in my eyes.

On our first visit, Divyansh had seen almost all the places in Israel except a southern port town, Elat, which, amongst other things, was known for coral life in the Red Sea. Sushil discussed the idea of visiting Elat with Savdas, who readily agreed to drive them there. So, they planned a visit to Elat by road. En route, they saw the picturesque Dead Sea and desert plantations. For the next two days, they completely forgot the mental turbulence caused by the recent medical complications and enjoyed the trip to the fullest. The photos Divyansh shared with me of his Elat trip also made me forget all his problems that I heard from Dr

Or a few days back. Bygones were bygones. For Divyansh, there was no hangover of the preceding days. Each day, he would take a fresh guard and move with new vigour. That's what they did in Elat, completely oblivious to all that Divyansh was going through.

> Now, as I stand at the precipice of this path,
> I truly understand,
> The true nature of transience, as it always is.

('Rebirth')

After returning from Elat, they met Dr Or who was ready with a treatment plan. The plan was to undergo certain medications for short-term benefit and certain others for long-term. The short-term medications were available in Mumbai and, therefore, he advised us to get them from Mumbai itself. But the long-term medication required was not available in India. Rather, no doctor in our country had the experience of administering the medicine. For that, Divyansh was advised to spend one month's time twice in Jerusalem with an interval of month. Dr Or revealed that the medicine had only recently been approved by the FDA after a successful trial. The caveat was that it was very expensive. Sushil didn't think too much and said he was ready to try everything for Divyansh. After this, they flew back to Mumbai for the short-term treatment under Dr Tapan Saikia.

After coming back from Jerusalem, Divyansh looked better. The recent nagging problems seemed to have disappeared. Sushil, without losing any time, put him under the care of Dr Tapan Saikia for the short-term treatment Dr Or had prescribed. He began to respond to the treatment and the test reports suggested improvement. In the midst of all these goings-on, Divyansh quickly finished the remaining entrance tests and was waiting for the results of the Class 12 board exams. What surprised me was his attempt to give CLAT, an entrance test for five-year courses in National Law School. When we discussed with him why amidst various engineering entrance tests, he chose to appear for admission in National Law School, he didn't say much. Then I remembered his career counselling we had done at Growth Centre, Chembur, by Ms Swati Salunkhe. She, in her report based on his assessment, commented that Divyansh would excel in all fields, be it engineering, medical science, commerce, law or even actuarial science. She had even remarked that the type of scores Divyansh had got after his assessment was rarely experienced by her team at the centre.

In the fourth week of May, the Class 12 board exam results were out. This time, too, Divyansh surprised us hugely. Before the results, I recollected the circumstances he was in after returning from Jerusalem while preparing for the examination. The highest result of education is tolerance and perseverance in the process. Divyansh comprehensively proved his success all through with his approach and the blueprint of preparation, which were immeasurable, unlike academic results in marks. Success is also peace of mind that results in self-satisfaction in knowing that one did one's best. People like Divyansh are never too concerned about what marks they might finally score. To me, Divyansh always demonstrated his detached attachment with the academic scores he got. This result was no different. To our surprise and also to the utter amazement of the teachers of KC College, Mumbai, where he studied, he was amongst the top five in the college in his stream. I was on top of the world to see his astounding success. This success too was earned bit by bit.

Now, the next good news. After the disaster of the JEE (Main), examination, he was successful in getting admission in a Narsee Monjee Trust-affiliated engineering college in Mumbai in his favourite discipline, Computer Science. Considering his need to study from a Mumbai-based college, this college was a decent one with good faculty and infrastructure. It was a cathartic moment for me where I could see him again succeed in the sense we normally mean. My wish for him to study Computer Science in Mumbai was partly fulfilled. The only difference was the college was not an IIT. In the competitive world we are in, a person like Divyansh needed a decent platform to showcase his talent. This college provided one to him.

One day, I received on my phone a ping for his Facebook status update. What was thought provoking to me was his Facebook profile bio. It stirred me completely. Though he had created his Facebook account a year back, this was the first occasion I could see his profile. The profile message read:

GET BUSY LIVING OR GET BUSY DYING.

It took me some time to realize what he meant by it. The words contained in the thought are few, but the message they convey is so profound that one would be tempted to know more about the person who made this his life motto. I have not an iota of doubt about how Divyansh practised and applied the thought in entirety in his life. This prompted me to check some of his earlier posts on his wall. My initial expectation was that his messages would be typical of a fledgling youth. Here again, I found his level of understanding and reflections on a multitude of issues on a different paradigm. There was a newspaper clipping with a photo of a doctor who had proudly got himself clicked with a new-born baby with a rare disorder. Divyansh responded to this by writing:

> I feel that what the doctor has done here is highly condemnable, so is the way he is holding that baby with a proud smile on his face. Just disgraceful, disgusting, insensitive and opportunist.
>
> In the last paragraph, the doctor talks about the rarity of this disorder. Well, even if it is so rare, parental consent is absolutely necessary before going ahead to take photos of the stricken infant. And maybe then can it be posted in

a medical journal. But circulate on social media and shout it out to the world? Just deplorable.

This is the common mentality I guess—stand on roads and watch a scuffle but not make any interference, anything abnormal? Well, let us go and see it? *Oh, dekh ye bachha kitna kaala/gora/mota/patlaa/ajeeb hai.* That insensitivity is what is on aggressive display here in this case.

It is only a saving grace that the baby passed on to a better realm in 3 days, otherwise the life it would live would be filled more with ignominy, shame, ostracization, nodding and disapproving faces than the medical support it might need.

The point that Divyansh was trying to drive home was that the implicit dignity of a patient and his/her parents needs to be respected and protected. Actions like this should be avoided as far as possible, and the least a doctor is expected to do is to refrain from indulging in it for cheap publicity at the cost of another's dignity. There was another message like this in response to a newspaper advertisement by a homecare specialist for cancer patients, wherein a cancer patient was depicted with bald head and in a frail condition crouched on a bed. The larger issue which invited his response was, should a cancer patient be portrayed as condemned like this? Is this the only identity left for a cancer patient? He wrote:

Despicable, deplorable, no words to describe this advertisement in *The Times of India* issue of today. If they really wanted to promote their brand, they could have done so in a better way rather than showing a person curled up in despair.

This just highlights the extent to which some can go to get to the top. The scare propaganda!

And I bet, this brand, or the newspaper for that matter,

doesn't care about the afflicted, doesn't care about their families, doesn't care about their trauma, but only looks for their money.

Who could have understood better than him the pain and the tribulations a patient goes through, and that too a cancer patient? It's not that Divyansh only decried such advertisements. He highly appreciated an advertisement by Jaslok Hospital, Mumbai, on treating a patient suffering from Parkinson's disease. The tagline of the advertisement was: 'In a Significant Global Medical Breakthrough, a Man Sips Tea'. Divyansh was so moved with the tag line evoking positivity that he wrote:

> This is how medical advertisements should be done... Subtle, yet powerful, and extremely empowering, to the sufferers and their kin alike.

The esoteric thought like respecting the dignity of a person, and especially that of a patient, should be understood and practised by one and all.

Divyansh began attending classes after taking admission in the engineering college. But the time was fast approaching when he had to travel to Jerusalem for undergoing the treatment for long-term benefit as suggested by Dr Or. Divyansh was a little reluctant to miss classes in the new college. Here, I must mention the name of pro vice-chancellor (VC) of the college, Mr S.Y. Mhaiskar, who encouraged Divyansh to prioritize his treatment. As for classes, he assured him that the respective teachers would post daily updates and assignments on the college website in the class group, which he could access from Jerusalem, read and solve. As far as his attendance was concerned, he assured him he need not worry. What a noble person he was. I bow in complete reverence to him.

10

DELICATE DREAMS, TREMBLING ARMS

The next issue to be resolved was who would accompany Sushil and Divyansh as they were to stay there for at least for a month, if not more. Sushil advised me to avoid going, lest Ananya would have to miss her classes for a long period. Anshoo was unavailable and so was Mridul because of their engagements in their offices and personal lives. There came another good samaritan, my younger sister Shikha (Meenu), who volunteered to go along and take care of Divyansh in my absence. The kind of relationship and camaraderie Shikha shared with Divyansh has already been discussed. It is to be noted that Shikha then had a five-year-old child whom she had to leave to the care of her husband Arvind, who was a commandant in the Central Industrial Security Force. Arvind readily agreed to let Shikha travel with Divyansh. It was a tough ask for a mother to leave a five-year-old child, that too for a month. Shikha did that. Her unpretentious love and affection for Divyansh was limitless. As a mother, I felt humbled to see her benevolence for us.

One more worrisome factor was the cost of the impending treatment which Dr Or had indicated would be high, as the medicine was newly approved after years of trial. As we were thinking of ways and means to arrange the funds required, Dr Or sent Sushil a mail mentioning that he had approached a German pharmaceutical company to supply this medicine free of cost for

Divyansh. Keeping in view Divyansh's background as Dr Or had written in his mail, the company agreed to supply it at no cost. Nobility has no boundary. It carries all the more value when it is done unassumingly. Dr Or, after their departure from Jerusalem, never indicated what he was up to as far as arranging this medicine was concerned. Sushil neither expected him to arrange it free of cost nor ever indicated this to him. All his life, whatever we did, was completely on our own strength and resources. But what made Dr Or arrange the medicine free of cost when we had not asked him to? The only answer we could find was probably the unique relationship which Divyansh shared with him, where a doctor and a patient seemed to have been transformed into ambassadors of noble humane acts and where an act like this is done as much for one's own intrinsic satisfaction as for the other's benefit.

Time appeared to be limping towards Divyansh's side. First, a good result in the Class 12 board examination, then admission in an engineering college in the subject he wanted and, finally, three hurdles in his travelling to Jerusalem—namely, missing lectures in college and attendance, who would accompany them and the cost of treatment—were smoothly sorted out. I would not say this was mere luck turning our tide. Since the past few years, I had stopped believing in a phenomenon like luck, and if at all it existed, it was not for us. Luck, as is said, is being in the right place at the right time. What was now happening with Divyansh, as I saw it, was a result of his inspiring persona where he was receiving all the right things in the right ways from the people whose lives he had touched, be it Mr Mhaiskar, Shikha, Dr Reuven Or or anyone else. That's the nuanced difference between luck and inspiration. All these events steadily began to germinate a long-embedded thought in me that Divyansh came into this life, and into our lives, with a purpose.

When Divyansh was diagnosed with this fresh round of complications after the transplantation, this time, Sushil and I decided not to inform our families about the latest developments. I always aspired to fill happiness in my parents' lives. I did too, on many occasions. But now, my father was retired, and I did not wish to let them go through another drill of mental agony for us. If I was not able to give them the happiness they deserved, at least I could save them from avoidable worries.

This time, too, they decided to stay in the same apartment in Jerusalem where we had stayed during the transplantation. The place was close to the hospital, clean and the staff was cooperative and, by then, known to us. They extended all possible support to make their stay comfortable. Dr Or, at the beginning of the treatment, was in Italy on a professional assignment. But he had ensured all arrangements for Divyansh for easy hospitalization and medication before he left. All the doctors of his team, namely, Dr Shapira, Dr Batia and Dr Segal, were given a clear brief and protocol of the treatment by Dr Or. This medication, which is a kind of immunotherapy, was being administered for the first time in the Hadassah Hospital and Divyansh became a pioneer patient to showcase the efficacy of this wonder-drug. The medicine was to be administered intravenously for 28 days continuously. Without any hitches, the treatment was started from the first week of July. Barring a few known side effects, Divyansh was able to tolerate the drug with ease. After a week, he was discharged from the hospital, strapping on a sling bag containing a small pump and a pouch of medicine connected to him through an IV line for its continuous administration. The sling bag became a body part of his for the next three weeks, which he had to carry even to the toilet or while taking a shower. Every third day, he had to go to the hospital for a refill of the medicine and follow-up. Divyansh's new life seemed to have begun in a new system, in which he did not allow anything to hinder what he wanted, be it his studies, an evening walk, going to the mall or attending get-togethers or dinner at Navdeep's and Savdas's homes. Much to our astonishment, he was able to pursue his college studies and assignments with remarkable ease. He remained in touch with his classmates regularly. More surprising was that many a time, he scored better marks than others in various assignments given by the teachers. He became an exemplar of the statement that engineering college studies can be so easy. Actually, that was not easy; Divyansh made it appear easy.

Meanwhile, Sushil had a rude shock of his life, and so did we all, when we received news that his father, who we all called Babooji, had to be hospitalized in Patna owing to certain medical complications. Though there were four of his brothers and their children to take care of him, Sushil felt the urgent need to visit him. While Sushil went through this mental turmoil, Babooji was shifted to the ICU in an emergency condition. In the next couple of days, he was put on life support for pneumonia. Sushil was completely at a loss. He was being tested morally. One the one hand, he had to take care of his son in Israel and, on the other, he desperately wanted to see his ailing father who was by then on the brink of death. The moral crisis he experienced was humungous. Divyansh sensed this and asked him to go to Patna, assuring him he would manage everything on his own. But it was not all that easy for Sushil. The drug which Divyansh was being administered had resulted in severe neurological storms in a few reported cases during trial stage. It was a possibility and Sushil was aware of it. Every day, Sushil called his brother in Patna for an update on Babooji's condition, which was worsening. He must have cried many times railing at why he was driven to this crossroad. Of all the six siblings, Sushil was the youngest in his family and closest to his father. Babooji died on the morning of 27 July. Sushil instantly decided to fly to Patna to attend his last rites. Navdeep Singh again came to our rescue. He not only managed his air tickets, but also assured him that he would take care of Divyansh round the clock in his absence. With his help,

Sushil first came to Mumbai and then together, we flew to Patna for Babooji's last rites. It was huge shock for all of us to lose both Sushil's parents within six months of each other. After the cremation, Sushil went back to Jerusalem, by which time Dr Or had returned from his trip. He seemed to be happy with Divyansh's progress. He planned his next round of treatment in the months of September–October. Sushil only came back with all of them after completion of the first round of treatment.

My family was reunited on 6 August, when Sushil, Divyansh and Shikha returned from Jerusalem.

While we were in Patna for Babooji's ceremonies, Divyansh was agitated with some political decision in Delhi and the administrative apathy to the cause of the needy. After a long three-month pause since he wrote 'Catharsis', he penned a poem 'The Power and the Powered'. Human governance in all its forms—democracy, autocracy, monarchy, dictatorship or primitive governance—has two distinctive facets, namely, those who govern and those who are governed. The former is vested with authority to rule in accordance with the law. But its authority cannot stand in isolation, unmindful of the concerns and aspirations of the subjects. Power always comes with embedded responsibility to ensure that subjects are governed in a just manner. But does this always happen? Can the powered and the powerful not be envisaged to exist in the right synergy, complementing the existence of each other? This is what he tried to articulate through this poem.

A long mane, grey with wisdom,
A stance speaking righteous,
Eyes filled with ethos,
He nods his head in dismay.

"Such a shame."
Are the sullen words,
Exhaled in the sigh,

He breathed out.
Power and Responsibility,
Are the inseparable brothers,
The powered rest upon whom,
Delicate dreams, and trembling arms.

The way Divyansh dived straight into his college curriculum after returning from Jerusalem, he seemed to have put his life on switch mode with remarkable ease. Attending classes, tutorials and seminars became his regular chores. There was neither any hangover of all that he went through in the past few months, nor was he was concerned about his remaining treatment in the months of September–October. To him, each moment of life was worth a year which he resolved to live to the maximum. If you can't live longer, live deeper. But what fascinated me was seeing his ever-increasing flock of friends. Gradually, his classmates knew more about him and became his admirers.

One day, Divyansh told Sushil about his desire to make forays into writing blogs in the digital space. So far, he had been writing poems. Now, he also wished to create his own dedicated blog wall where he could reflect his thoughts. In order to procure his own space, he had to pay a subscription fee by credit card. Sushil happily encouraged Divyansh in his novel thought. I wondered what he would write about first; he invariably came up with dynamic new thoughts and their perfect execution. Apart from writing, the two passions closest to his heart were food and music. Can food and music have a striking similarity? Only a passionate person like Divyansh would venture into writing about it because he had assimilated food and music in layers. Thus, the first piece he wrote on his blog wall, http://divyanshatman.blog, his 'Literary Whetstone', on 17 September 2016 was 'Mellifluous Music and Moreish Meals'. The reflection was so abstract yet thought-provoking that one would look at music and food differently after reading his blog. He wrote:

There are few things that offer intangibles to people as profound as music. And food.

While both may be different in terms of fathomable appearance, food of course being a physical spread on a plate, and music being something you 'listen to', the perceptible organization and 'experience giving mechanism' of both, is the same. Let me elucidate this.

Every piece of music has the bass section, which forms the foundation of the music piece. The bass section comprises partly of the percussion, the cello/the bass guitar/double bass, and other such instruments, which have a heavy baritone and stay in the background on which the other parts of the piece are built upon. Remove this, and the piece loses its impact. In fact, it has been found that the bass section of a symphony is significantly responsible for eliciting and creating 'emotion records' in the human brain, which enable us to create preferences in our playlist. So the inviting hard thump and groove that you hear coming from a concert some distance away that makes you feel part of it is a very integral part of any musical piece.

The same goes for food. Let me give you a very simple example. Consider a pizza (like how you would in a mathematical proof). The pizza dough, baked into a crust, forms the base, both literally and figuratively for the rest of the pizza to go on. Literally, well, you cannot just have the cheese and toppings if you don't have something chunky to bite into. You could, but the 'satisfaction factor' will just not be there. The dish as a whole won't make sense. And figuratively, the richness and creaminess of the cheese, the tartness and tanginess of the sauce, and the astute and distinct textures of the topping, all need a 'neutral' but robust foundation, on which they can choreograph their dance, performed on the palate. This correlation can be applied to any type of dish.

Then comes the rhythm section. The percussion (drums, tabla, etc.) set the pace and pulse for the musical piece. They dictate how the music will flow, where it will pick pace, where it will slow down, where the cadence will rise and fall. They are like the route navigators for the car that is the musical piece.

In food, it is the salad and patty in the sandwich, the cheese and marinara base on the pizza or the texture of the noodles in the stir fry. These set the tone and form a main part of the body of what you are eating. They define the flavours that will burst in your mouth, and into your sinus and throat, creating palpitations for spicy, ripples on the tongue for tangy and tart, chill in case of cold and icy, warm and ticklish in case of umami and so on. The list could go on and on, just like the rhythmic variations do.

The vocals come in next. They stand on top of the pedestal created by the bass and rhythm sections and are the limelight of the performance. They are the ones in the driving seat, powered on by the car's various parts. They are the 'interpreters' that give literal form to the abstract feelings elicited by the instrumentation and orchestration.

The toppings on your pizza, the add-ons in your sandwich, the distinct taste in your soup, the sweetness of your gelato, the roasted flavour in your coffee are the singers translating the clefs, brieves, quavers, minims, crotchets of the dish into your gastronomical senses.

The treble and bass sections top it off, providing the occasional and required high points and trills that zap you into a high every time it occurs in the symphony. They do not have a presence throughout the musical piece, maybe at the start, or at the end, and a few times in between.

That dash of fresh basil and rosemary on your al dente pasta, the sprinkle of oregano and Tabasco on your pizza, the fresh coriander on your daal, the nutty sesame seeds on your baked goodies or the tart pickle you dig into with every mouthful are what fall into the treble section of food, cutting and cleansing their way across distinct shades of flavours and textures.

Music and food are the siblings who have different physical and characteristic outlooks, but similar intrinsic traits imbibed from upbringing by the same parents—they may look different, and have different personas, but the underlying soul in both is the same. And both are excellent mediums of creating and nurturing harmony, tranquillity, humanity and unity among us humans.

I did not know music and food could be compared so vividly and convincingly. What an imagination to think that music and food are siblings which are mediums of nurturing and creating harmony and uniting humans!

11

DON'T LET THIS MASK
BE YOUR MASTER

Third week of September, 2016: time to go to Jerusalem for the second round of immunotherapy. Again, who would accompany them? The thought was on my mind since they had returned in August after round one. It was very frustrating for me not to be able to travel with Divyansh because of Ananya's schooling. Sushil was a constant in all his travels and treatment. I was craving to do my part. My youngest sister Shivangi came to our help. She took leave from her office for a month and happily agreed to travel and help them in treatment and daily chores in the apartment. With the help of Dr Or, her visa for Israel was made in no time.

This time, Dr Or was available from day one to take care of his treatment. All our friends, namely, Navdeep Singh, Savdas, Leuma and her husband Gideon, Michelle, Soshi and Caron, came forward to help them and often invited them for dinner in turns. The treatment began smoothly. The hospitalization in the first week and the treatment for the remaining three weeks was continued from home with the same sling bag containing the pouch of medicine to be administered intravenously 24X7 for three weeks with the help of a pump. In this trip, Divyansh was remarkably in full throttle on his literary sojourn and delivered three poems back to back, all evoking his novel thoughts, while undergoing treatment. The pump in his sling bag, it seemed, was not just pumping medicine into his body but also boosting his thoughts.

Divyansh disliked pretentious behaviour. However, he never expressed it in either his action or words. As Lord Shaftesbury said, 'After all, the most natural beauty in the world is honesty and moral truth; for all beauty is truth.' Taking it further, if someone is honest, then why he would indulge in pretentious behaviour? Divyansh not only practiced honesty but also ensured he did it with right action. This thought inspired him to write his next poem, 'The Mask' on 21 September 2016. The reason I write dates against each of his poems has a thought behind it, which I will explain as I progress. Here are some excerpts of this poem:

Some wear it to hide,
The darkness and maliciousness trapped inside,
Feeding this ever-growing inferno,
Through genuine, 'gleaming' smiles,
Visible to the world,
As an amiable, warm shine.
Shining extremely bright on the surface,
Casting shadows of pitch black jealousy within,
On sensing happiness and good fortune of others,
Yearning wickedly, with extreme ominous desire,
For its conversion,
Into eternal misfortune.

...

Don't let this mask be your master,
Make it your apprentice,
Use it as a shining diamond, if you have to,
Emanating your true persona, far and wide,
And not as a genie lamp,
To trap the true you,
That ought be out.

Some people wear a mask to cover their darker and unholy side. However, there are people who also wear such masks for other reasons—to hide their pain and vulnerability for fear of unwanted pity from others. In both cases, it is the mask which becomes our master and guides us to exhibit conditioned behaviour.

But why do we need such masks?
Why wear them?
Let's show the world the real in us…
Good or Bad.

The time spent at home that Divyansh cherished the most was always when he sat with us as we sipped our morning tea in the extended area of the living room, which overlooked the Arabian Sea. Normally, that was the time we were in a relaxed mood and discussed lighter topics. He must have observed the texture of my discussions with Sushil and the ever-strengthening conjugal bond with him over the years. Divyansh was a keen observer and noted how our animated and light-hearted discussions used to set the mood of the day. For him, a 'cuppa' became a metaphor symbolizing romanticism and the growing warmth between a husband and a wife. He put down his thoughts in the poem titled 'The "Cupple"' on 26 September 2016, just five days after he had written 'The Mask'. The title of the poem is a word coined by him, and as one reads the poem, the subtle meaning conveyed through this word becomes profound. This is what he said:

Meet the "Cupple"—
Arriving with swagger—
The charming, dynamic, flamboyant
Mr Cocoa Robusta,
And clutching his arm,
Sauntering in the most dainty of ways,
The demure, the bedazzling,
Mrs Flora Foliage.

...

The "Cupple"—
Are the heralds of the day,
Giving an encouraging push,
To conquer the new day,
Gently lullabying the yawning, and sprouting laze.

On reading this poem, Dr Archana, his friend Dhruv's mother, wrote, 'After reading "The 'Cupple'", I started seeing my cup of tea in a new light. Thanks Divyansh for infusing such a breath of fresh ideas.'

I was very happy to see Divyansh delivering so many thought-provoking poems so frequently.

The life of a woman and her journey, from being a baby to her childhood, then adulthood, culminating in wedlock, which finally gives birth to motherhood, requires a thoughtful mind to unravel it, layer by layer. Just four days after he wrote 'The "Cupple"', Divyansh came out with another brilliant poem titled 'She' on 30 September 2016 to celebrate the various colours of womanhood. The closest woman in Divyansh's life was I, through whom he could probe so much to decode various facets of womanhood, which, paradoxically, I couldn't. It looked more appreciable and inconceivable as it came from a person who was hardly 19 years old. This is 'She':

She has seen a lot,
In this drama called life,
Cared for, loved deeply,
By the generation she is the seed of.

Sitting in her cradling chair,
Sighs impregnated with fulfilment,
Vision reflecting contentment,
She looks into her husband's eyes.

A mystical communication, devoid of words ensues,
As they clutch their throbbing hands,
Ready to face,
The transient whim of change,
Accepting heart fully,
The inevitable nature of imminence.

Three big poems, all with different and not much ravelled milieu, in just nine days... why was he in a hurry to fill his basket of poetry? All this, whilst he was undergoing immunotherapy with disturbing side effects. While I struggled to find the answer to this question, he wrote another thought stimulating piece on his blog wall 'Remember the Human...'. The opening five lines summed up well the message he intended to convey. Worth quoting are those inspiring lines:

'Are you Hindu or Muslim?'
'I am hungry...'

A simple, two-line conversation. So brief, yet so powerful, encompassing such a deep message, and bringing forth the moot question: Is religion above humanity?

I could see his soul reflected like a flowing river, possessing pristine water, and enamouring a person like me, filling me with a new sense of wisdom as it moved from one rapid to another. Ironically, a mother was learning from her 19-year-old son about the niceties of life.

While Divyansh was undergoing treatment in Jerusalem, back in Mumbai, I was busy getting the new flat Sushil was allotted by the government ready. This flat was spacious and located in a serene place. The idea was to shift there by the beginning of December. Divyansh, Sushil and Shivangi returned to Mumbai on 20 October. Dr Or advised Divyansh to come once more around Christmas for three days of follow-up.

Since their return from Jerusalem, I was generally happy

because I could see Divyansh happy and we were soon going to shift into a new, bigger and well-located flat. The three big festivals, namely, Dussehra, Diwali and Chhath, fell soon after their arrival, and Divyansh's much-improved condition added zest to their celebration. The most difficult festival for us to celebrate had always been Chhath where one has to fast for three days. I had started performing Chhath Puja since 2010, after Divyansh was diagnosed with leukaemia for the first time. It was my penance to propitiate Chhath Mata while performing Arghya to the Sun God for Divyansh's well-being. It was also true that of all the festivals, performing Chhath was closest to my heart. I used to wait for this festival to arrive. I always conjured a healthy life for Divyansh through this puja. Chhath and Divyansh became synonymous for me. Divyansh too loved the fact that I was doing the Chhath Puja for him. He always accompanied me through all the rituals and held my hands when I stepped into the sea/river to offer Arghya. It was he from whose hand I drank water, looking at each other to break my three days of fasting.

This time, we celebrated Chhath forgetting whatever happened with Divyansh in the past and wished Chhath Mata to grant him good health as I offered Arghya to the Sun God at sunset and sunrise. The best penance is to have patience with the sorrow God permits. I had been keeping my patience since 2009. It was seven long years of Divyansh's teen life. My well of patience seemed dried up now. It wailed as I bowed down to the Sun God in complete reverence at sunset and sunrise.

Since Divyansh came back, he again switched himself completely to the college curriculum. His friends were waiting for him to add an element of wisdom to their classroom. One day, he discussed with his father the menacing onslaught of the ISIS, and in the same breath, the growing Hindu fundamentalism, though its effect was felt only at the fringe level. After their intense discussion, Divyansh wrote a thought-provoking article on his blog wall, 'A World without Religion'. Suffice it to quote an extract about how a young man of 19 years had envisioned the meaning of religion in the emerging world order.

> Can't we live and thrive in a world devoid of religion? A world where humanity, kindness, unity, love, righteousness, dignity are the values that form the alternative to religion. A truly egalitarian society devoid of any stereotypes, discrimination or profiling. A society where International Health Day, Men's Day, Women's Day, Son's day, Daughter's Day, Mother's Day, Teacher's Day, Father's Day, World Peace Day, World Environmental Day and so on are celebrated with as much gusto as religious festivals are. A world that still worships God, but without the various checkpoints required to meet Him/Her. A world that is not God-fearing, but God-loving.
>
> ...
>
> God created man, as those having faith say. But after that, never revealed His identity to him. So, man, since time immemorial, has been constantly searching for Him. In doing that, his mortal mind carved various paths, filled with sharp curves, steep bends and speed bumps, for the realization of the Supreme Being. Now those paths are coming at loggerheads, and man is nowhere close to his destination. Why not remove all these roads and 'message' Him whenever and wherever we want, if He is omnipresent, or, in the digital age, 'always online'? I don't think God would want His creation to destroy itself or suffer in His pursuit. Any creator wouldn't want that to happen to his creation.

Years later, this particular blog was published in a magazine of a leading school in Panchagani.

As advised by Dr Or, Divyansh and Sushil went to Jerusalem

for the last follow-up in December around Christmas. The trip was planned for only three days, so it was not necessary for me to accompany them. Divyansh was found fine after his check-up. It was a festive time in Israel with the celebration of Hanukkah. This festival commemorates the triumph of the Jews over the Greek rulers. Its sanctity derives from the spiritual aspect of their victory and is observed for eight days. The central feature of this festival is the lighting of candles each evening: one on the first day, two on the second and so on. The city of Jerusalem was in full glow with its festivity. After the check-up, Dr Or invited Divyansh and Sushil to dinner at his home to celebrate this festival with them on the eighth day of Hanukkah. As before, despite his busy schedule, Dr Or came to pick them up from their apartment in the evening and drove them to his home on the fringe of the city. He had invited some other guests as well, and they celebrated the last day of the festival with real gusto. Following others, Divyansh also lit candles to celebrate the spiritual aspect of his victory over leukaemia. Dr Or took personal care of Divyansh and Sushil as most of the others were conversing in Hebrew. So that they should not feel left out, he translated all the Hebrew discussions for them. Divyansh had told me that day was chilling cold and yet, Dr Or didn't hesitate to drive them back to their apartment at midnight.

Spiritual aspect of victory? Well, the spiritual evolution of Divyansh became more profound after he came back. As for his victory over leukaemia, his spiritual growth actually dwarfed its significance. I realized that much later.

12

HERE WE GO AGAIN

'Hello, this is Dr Saikia. Unfortunately, Divyansh has again been diagnosed with CNS relapse. The CSF test result has just been seen by me. At this stage, I would not like to expose him to any more treatment. Actually, there are no more treatment options left for him now. Let him now live his life till...'

'What are you saying, Dr Saikia? Relapse, I can understand. But please think from the perspective of a father. How can he leave his son to battle without treatment? Like my son, I would also like to fight till...'

After returning from Kolkata, where Sushil and I had gone to visit the Dakshineshwar Temple to take the blessings of Goddess Kali Maa for Divyansh's healthy life, the episodes of intermittent threatening headaches coming to him never stopped. Rather, they were worsening. Divyansh's second semester examination of his engineering college was round the corner. He was pulling on with his studies despite all physical difficulties. Seeing no end to his nagging physical discomfort, Sushil took him to Dr Tapan Saikia, his oncologist in Mumbai, for assessment and advice. We were aware that Dr Saikia had been insisting on getting Divyansh's medical assessment done considering recent events, which we were planning for after his exams. Ultimately, we had to give in. First an MRI, then a PET CT scan and finally a CSF test led Divyansh back to the same path he had been treading for long. Yes, it was the same issue that had occurred before transplantation: leukaemic relapse in the CNS. Dr Saikia was a conservative doctor who practised medicine with ethics. He professed that a patient should not be exposed to unnecessary medication if it didn't ameliorate him or her for even a short term. According to him, Divyansh had reached a stage where all types of available treatments, including BMT, were tried on him, and even after all this, the disease had returned. He was quite blunt in saying to Sushil that day on the phone that he had been practising oncology for nearly 40 years, and based on his experience, he believed that a time had come now to stop giving any treatment to Divyansh. It was easier for a doctor to say this, but could parents remain mute in the face of it? I looked at Divyansh; I was sure he understood what was going on. This time, the feeling of despondency was visible on his face. He was crestfallen. With tears in his eyes, he said to me, 'I have been bearing with my nightmare for years. I didn't ever complain of it. Now, I get a feeling that time is trying to bulldoze me with its brute force. I am being tested for my patience and perseverance. Even that has a limit.' Hearing this, all I could do in answer to his emotional outburst was hug him tightly, weeping inconsolably till he wiped my tears and made me rest on the bed. I went to his room after an hour and surprisingly found his demeanour well-composed. It seemed he was getting himself ready to fight one more battle. He gulped a paracetamol and got busy with his studies.

To treat malignancy in the CNS, there is only one medicine, Methotrexate, which is injected intrathecally, that is, through the spine. There are very few medicines that can cross the blood–brain barrier for the treatment of the spread of malignancy in the brain system. Radiation, another treatment option in such cases, was not considered advisable in Divyansh's case, as he had already been exposed to it before transplantation and further exposure would cause irreversible toxicity in the brain.

Sushil fell back on tried-and-tested Dr Or to discuss any promising treatment option. Dr Or was of the view that Divyansh needed a few doses of Methotrexate immediately, till he could find any treatment option available globally, even if that was in the trial stage. He talked to Dr Saikia and convinced him to begin giving him Methotrexate for his immediate remission. By that time, Dr Saikia probably realized his error in the curt manner of giving his opinion to Sushil. That was 14 March 2017, I distinctly remember. Many things were happening that day. Around 8.30 p.m., Dr Saikia texted Sushil: 'My sincere apologies. I couldn't behave differently. It breaks my heart, but I am a human being too. Can't act like a machine when I know what we are looking at. I am always here to help him suffer less.'

He then called Sushil and advised him to bring Divyansh the next day to begin treatment with Methotrexate, as advised by Dr Or. From the discussion with the doctors, we also realized that this treatment would give him but short reprieve. So we hectically began looking for a long-term solution in collaboration with Dr Or, by consulting various other treatment centres internationally. 14 March, however, ended on a high note. As I have emphasized time and again, Divyansh possessed some divine spirit to combat adversities like this with utmost poise, and in the process, he would help us tide over the crises. This day was no different. At about 9 p.m., after dinner, he sat at the study table. I thought he was preparing for the examination, mindfully mindless of what was happening to him. By 10.30 p.m., he was done with his studies. The study he had done was not for the exam but of the finer nuances of tiding over the crisis at hand. He wrote a poem that day titled 'Here We Go Again', which he wrote not only for himself, but also for us. The excruciating pain, both physical and mental, on the relapse of leukaemia was being successfully harnessed into constructive energy, which was apparent from his pleasant countenance. Yes, the endless suffering caused by the pain was visible through the radiance of his face. He was celestially composed, which gave us impetus, enough to carry on uninhibited through the daunting path ahead. The inspiring poem which became quite popular in days to come evoked courage and optimism.

'Here We Go Again' described the profoundness of self-belief. In the 'game of patience', as the erudite Divyansh called it, we should invoke ourselves to raise our spirit so high as to enable us to foresee triumph towards the end. Triumph, as envisioned by him, was not and could not be only an end result but also meant how we carried on with this battle. I am quoting this entire poem: only then can its profoundness be felt.

Here we go again,
You and me, facing each other,
Time, the untiring witness,
Sighing and gazing;
Who blinks first.

Long has this lasted,
An entire boyhood;
While we go on and on.
Staring are the unrelenting countenances,
Into the abyss of transience

Pretty impressive is your motivation,
Pulling me, pushing me down at will.
There come times, the well of patience when,
Seems parched in front of your presence.

Save your breath, save your energy,
Desist from these fool-hardys,
No despair, no maelstrom of yours,
Terrifies me, jitters me.
Not anymore.

You see, I have become the master,
Of the storm you so well orchestrate,
Right up my alley, bursting at my sleeves,
Are contemplations, you plot next.

It is a game of patience,
Naked, languid stares,
Where the triumphant will be me,
Laughing at your soreness.

We can play this game as long as you wish,
Until you let yourself to ruin,
I will continue to stare,
At your crumbling will.

The motivation conveyed through 'Who blinks first' was enough for us to end an otherwise turbulent day with a high spirit. Paradoxically, all through his never-ending battle with his nemesis, we, as parents, treaded the path shown by our *son* who was still in his teens. There was not an iota of doubt about Divyansh leading us from the front. That day, too, was no different.

Karmanyewadhikaraste Ma Phaleshu Kadachana !

We have control only on our karma or duty, not on the fruits it will finally bear. Divyansh internalized this thought profoundly, and reflected it through his evoking actions.

The next day, Divyansh was to be hospitalized for a day for the administration of Methotrexate under the care of Dr Saikia. He had to perform another karma on that day: practical for the second semester examination. He told us to keep a bed in the hospital ready and that he would reach there straightaway after finishing his practical exam. He also advised me to look for a single room in the hospital so that he could study at night. I was completely in awe at the way he epitomized the karma theory of life. When he reached the hospital from college, he nonchalantly told me that he had shared news of the relapse with his class friends and assured them that he would be back soon. I remembered the letter he had written after transplantation from Jerusalem on my birthday in 2015, where he had mentioned 'missing the tender touch' in his treatment process. I didn't want to deprive him of this anymore. For the first time in his entire treatment process, I decided to play my part actively. I would now become a mother donning the avatar of a nurse, who would take care of his medical needs, lacing my care with a tender touch. So, even the next day, thanks to Divyansh, was a fulfilling one—the day he finished his practical exams, knowing full well that he might have to miss the theory papers in all probability. Besides, it was heartening to see Dr Saikia in action again for the intrathecal administration of Methotrexate to him, which, after 2–3 doses, would bring a short-term remission till a lasting treatment option was found.

I wanted to share Divyansh's latest developments with Raji Madam, our yoga teacher, with whom Divyansh was very close. I called her to convey the latest trauma of her Chhota Hanuman. After listening, she said she would get back to us soon, but she never did. I felt very hurt. The people we could count on to share our misery were few, she was one of them. Not hearing from her again after knowing our latest ordeal shook my self-respect. I felt dejected. Seeing this happening to me, Divyansh texted me the following message:

Mummy,

People will keep coming in and going out of our lives, Mummy. We have to choose how we deal with them. One, we can avoid all and just go on, walking along.

Two, we can choose to be influenced by what they say and then weigh where we want to head.

Three, we can appreciate all the good they bring to us, ignoring all the bad, or what they don't, feel happy at the little bit of concern they show, but refuse to be dependent on them and move ahead.

I suggest that you, me Papa, Ananya, we should all take these as their personal attributes, where we eliminate the chance of ever being hurt or cheated because of someone else.

Remember, maximum work in a reversible process in the thermodynamics of life.

The message gave me the insight to look within myself and regain my composure.

What about Anshoo's wedding? Should it be postponed? No, not at all. I was absolutely clear about it, though I had dreamt a lot about his wedding. The matter was discussed with us by Anshoo's father, and we advised him against the wedding's postponement. I realized, more so after learning the karma theory from Divyansh, that one is responsible for one's action and duty. Whether to go ahead with the wedding or not at that stage should have been guided by their own karma. We did our karma when the question was put before us. After that, it completely rested on theirs. I never wanted Anshoo to become a victim of our pain at the best time of his life. That's why I made sure to go along with him to the showroom for the final trial of his sherwani before we left for a place where Dr Or would advise us for Divyansh's treatment. Finally, all preparations for his wedding moved on as per plan. Here, we were preparing to embrace a new challenge in our lives in an alien country.

I remembered a call from Ajay on 1 January 2017. Ajay, who lived in New Jeresy, USA, was the husband of Sushil's cousin, Kavita, and worked there as a scientist at a big corporate. He had called us to wish us for the new year. He had heard a lot about Divyansh through common relatives. He casually advised us to explore the possibility of bringing Divyansh to USA to pursue his studies from there. We told him it had been Divyansh's long-cherished dream to study at MIT, but at that stage, the fruition of that dream looked like a remote possibility. But why did he propose this out of nowhere on that day? Was there any grand design in the offing?

Meanwhile, Dr Reuven Or called to inform us that there was a trial treatment in Texas, USA, which he thought held some promise. By then, Divyansh had achieved remission due to the administration of Methotrexate. Dr Or coordinated with a doctor of that hospital for Divyansh, and an appointment was fixed for 5 April 2017. The US Consulate in Mumbai was kind enough to grant us emergency visas. The deck was clear for us to fly to USA to explore a new life for Divyansh.

It was evident by then that Divyansh was going to miss his semester examination. The pro-VC, Mr Mhaiskar, again came to our rescue with a promise to hold another examination for Divyansh whenever he returned, so that he didn't have to miss a year on account of that. The initial plan was to stay there for a month and a half for the trial treatment.

Lately, whenever I faced adverse situations in life, more, related to Divyansh, I would often wish for Mridul to be by my side. And he would always be at my beck and call. Over a period of time, we mattered so much to him that he would notice even the slightest pain in my voice on phone calls. This time, too, while I was talking to him, he sensed my disturbed mental state. I had to tell him about the developments of the past few days. He didn't think even for a minute and decided to come to Mumbai the very next day from Dubai. He stayed with us for a couple of days and generally tried his best to lift our sagging mood. Before leaving for Dubai, he texted Divyansh:

> Whenever I leave you, especially in times like these, I always leave with a very heavy heart and it was so this time as well, but this time, there was one major difference. There

is absolutely no denying that nobody could have handled better the things that you have handled previously and until now, but earlier, I would still feel that there was a part you which wanted answers to some questions. However, for the first time, I felt a calmness in you that is almost terrifying to see in a young boy like yourself. On the one hand, this calmness is driving some calmness in everybody, on the other, as Papa rightly mentioned, it makes us want to tell you to share whatever you are feeling with us.

Trust me, there isn't a thing in this world that we can tell you to make you feel all right, to make us feel all right, and whatever we say would probably be a repetition, a rhetoric. Truth is, we, especially you, are chosen to go through all this and we all hate it but we have to go through this. Probably the only solace is that you have become a stronger, more hardened warrior and probably more equipped than anybody else to fight this, and I know that no matter the ordeal, you will come out of all this a winner, defeating destiny, defeating God's injustice.

Because more than God, more than anyone else, I now have faith in your strength. Love you and take care.

Divyansh replied:

Well, the only thing I could think of after reading your comment is the law of diminishing returns. Repeat too much of a rare occurrence, and it stops bothering you as it might have the first time.

The thing is, I have virtually seen myself going through this for so long, and through so many different ways, that there wasn't anything new to expect now. Like I said, as long as there is a way ahead, I am content.

Yes, it is pretty frustrating to go through it again and again and again and again, but that is not something in my hands, best I can probably do is not let this get to my mind.

Time and again, you come back to support me during my trying times, you came just when I needed you the most, and this is something that makes you one of the most 'essentials' for me.

Thank you, and cheers!

13

LET'S SEE WHAT YOU 'HAVE IN STORE' FOR ME

Life is known for its uncertainties. One's priorities change with time and situations. Probable makes way for the improbable. So, there is continuous interplay of one's priorities on the broad canvas of life. It is up to us how we adapt ourselves and allow them to interplay and flow with it. The essence of life lies in the enrichment it gets while priorities interplay. This is what Divyansh reflected when he wrote his next poem titled 'Priority's Play' on 29 March 2017, just two days before our travel to USA. Here is an excerpt from the poem:

An inquisitive child it is,
Let it play.
Beat and shape it the toddler will,
Into a masterpiece,
Of sense, and rationale.

Time had been the relentless testimony of Divyansh's adeptness while priorities in his life interplayed. This time, it was no different. We, too, followed him in imbibing this virtue.

For the first time ever, I was going to leave Ananya to live without me. She was hardly 15 years old then. We couldn't take her to USA as her exams were going on. My parents came home to stay in Mumbai and to take care of her in our absence. Full credit to Ananya for understanding my need to accompany Divyansh to USA to take care of him whilst he underwent treatment there. There was neither any whisper of a complaint as to how she would manage without me, nor any sadness visible on her face. In the past few months when Divyansh was looking good, we had decided to give undivided attention to her studies and personal care. Unfortunately, she needed to wait more for this.

When we decided to fly to USA, the plan was to stay at Ajay's home in New Jersey for three days and then move from there to Texas for the treatment.

We were off to USA on 31 March 2017.

> Let's see what You "have in store" for me
> For the ball is in Your court

('Catharsis')

Ajay and his wife Kavita lived in a sprawling bungalow in Burgan County, New Jersey. The bungalow was picturesquely located where the Passaic River flowed by the side of its lush green backyard. The layout of its living space was in duplex form, the living area and the kitchen were located on the ground floor and the bedrooms, upstairs. The walkway from the main gate leading to the bungalow was flanked by grass carpets on both sides, typical of the famous savanna grassland of the temperate region of USA. Ajay's office was located just across the river, at a driving distance of hardly five minutes. They had two pretty daughters, one almost of Divyansh's age, and the younger one, then a student of Grade 12 in a nearby school.

I met Ajay the first time then, though I had met Kavita once, a year back. Sushil too was meeting them after years that were hardly punctuated by any significant communication between them. They appeared very affable and warm and wanted to help us on all counts. Except for my own parents' and in-laws' homes, we hardly ever stayed in other relatives' homes when we were in their cities, just to avoid burdening them from hosting us.

This was the first time we were staying at a relative's home. The idea cemented when Ajay pestered Sushil to stay with them en route to Texas. He wanted to spend some time with us and meet Divyansh. Instinctively, I was reluctant at the very idea of being their guest even for a few days and I discussed my reservations with Sushil about it before we travelled. But considering there was no direct flight to Texas from Mumbai, we had to first go to Newark in New Jersey, and from there, catch another flight to our final destination. So, respecting Ajay's earnest request to stay with them, I changed my mind. As for Kavita, it needs to be mentioned that she was very close to Sushil's late father and my father-in-law, and this fact also led us to change our mind. She was seeing Divyansh for the first time, and as we entered her home, her first remark was that Divyansh was a mirror image of his grandfather, more specifically, his smile was like his grandfather's.

Struggling with bad jet lag that made us sleep through the day, we effectively began conversing only by the evening. They already knew a lot about Divyansh. We talked about the events of his past years and his academic and literary excellence amidst all this. Now came the big idea from Ajay's side which made me realize why Divyansh's recent medical problem led us there. The flying time from Mumbai to New Jersey was a long 16 hours as it was a direct flight. We had discussed with Divyansh the issue of how he would continue his studies in Mumbai when there was no viable treatment option left for him in the city. It would be difficult to pursue studies in Mumbai and continue taking treatment in USA. After the latest relapse, we were made to believe that there was only one treatment option, that too in a trial stage, available only in USA. We were concerned for his future. At this point, Ajay suggested that Divyansh should try for admission in an engineering college in USA in the coming fall semester by preparing for SAT and TOEFL, which he could do alongside his forthcoming treatment in Texas. Hearing this, I began joining various dots. Ajay called us out of the blue on 1 January and threw the idea of Divyansh's treatment and studies in USA. Then the relapse happened, and we were told the only treatment available was in USA. And finally, despite my reservations, we stayed with them en route to Texas. Actually, the first dot dated back to the year 2013, when Divyansh expressed his wish to study in USA after finishing his Class 10 board examination. It is said that your fate sometimes makes you laugh. The catch lies in discerning the reason for the laughter. All this could not have been coincidence. All these events had a common thread which I began unravelling as days passed. Were there some more dots this thread had to connect? Only time would tell. I felt we were ordained to flow like this by Divyansh's destiny. Obviously, we were quite receptive to Ajay's ideas. Divyansh, by that time, also realized that if at all he had any chance to make something of his life, it was going to be in USA. By the end of the next day, Ajay brought study materials for him to prepare for SAT and TOEFL. Divyansh promised to give it a serious try, though I was not sure how he would manage his study with the impending trial treatment and its side effects.

Before we left for Texas, Ajay and Kavita took us to the famous Times Square in New York City. We all were seated in the open rooftop of the tourist bus for sightseeing. Divyansh and Ajay sat separately in a corner, engrossed in serious discussion on educational opportunities available in USA and how Divyansh could make his future by studying there. Over a very short period of time, the kind of connection Ajay established with Divyansh was beyond my imagination. Ajay was genuinely invested in furthering Divyansh's interest in USA and, for that, he was ready to extend all possible help. Was Ajay's coming into Divyansh's life a part of the divine design?

As the bus passed the UN headquarters, I saw Divyansh look at it in a thoughtful mood. I was reminded about an event this January, when Divyansh took part in a MUN (Model United

Nations) staged in his college wherein he had represented Israel. Divyansh knew about Israel and its various problems due to his past visits. He was so happy after making his deliberation on Israel on that day. It was his token gesture to pay back what Israel had given to him. When he came home, he shared his MUN ID card of him as a representative of Israel with Dr Or, who was very happy to see that. Divyansh had told me that someday he would like to visit the UN office. Today, he was right at its doorstep. Sitting in the bus, he was possibly wondering when he might go inside to see its magnificent General Assembly hall. After the sightseeing bus tour, we spent a lot of time on the streets of Times Square, which are considered tourists' delight. The spark and gleam I saw in Divyansh's eyes were not from uneasiness caused by the CNS relapse or nervousness about the upcoming treatment. His eyes gleamed because he could see his promising future there. He was blazing one more time, foreseeing that the promising future Ajay talked about was achievable.

A day before our travel to Texas, Divyansh wrote a thought titled 'The Bass' on his blog. The 'bass' he referred to was the bass guitar he played. Music has no relevance if it doesn't impact us emotionally or mentally. That's why we often hear terms like soulful singing or rendition. Likewise, a musical masterpiece is created with the individual contribution of each instrument in creating the piece. One of the most important amongst them is the bass guitar, which lays the foundation of the composition, in the absence of which the musical composition would lose its soul. With this principle in mind, he began to explore the bass in our own lives, on whose foundation we built and owed our existence to. Some excerpts are as follows:

> Every musical piece is an intricate interplay of three very distinct components, dictating all the various parameters that define the feel, look and vibe of the piece. Essential among these components is the bass section—the section

that provides the foundation on which the proverbial 'architecture and masonry' of the symphony is done.

...

Are we also the bass in someone's life?

Knowingly or unknowingly, we do become [so]. The easiest relation to explain this would be the relationship between siblings—always [on] each other's lookout, dynamically evolving, morphing into a friend, an ear, an adviser, a perspective, a channel: unjudging, understanding, unconditional, unbiased.

Do you genuinely feel happy and rejoice when you see a dear/close one do well, excel, succeed in any of the endeavours he/she sincerely pursues? Do you find your happiness in their happiness? Well, you are the bass here then!

Like the way it is, finding good bass musicians who have established themselves to standards aspirants look is not a regular occurrence. There are only a handful of them who can be considered as 'A-Listers'.

Being the bass in someone's life isn't easy either. But strives can always be made.

Remember, there are a lot of people who form the bass to the musical piece—your life.

What a novelty of imagination in finding the metaphorical presence of a musical instrument in the web of relationships we weave for our existence!

14

BLOOD IS THICKER THAN WATER BUT SOME ARE THINNERS LIKE ASPIRIN

When we landed in Texas, Khush was at the airport to receive us and take us to the apartment he had hired for our stay. Khush is Shikha's husband Arvind's older brother who works in California. When he heard of our plan to visit there for treatment, he booked us an apartment near the hospital, paid the advance and remained available for us on the day we arrived by flying a long distance from California. Not just that, he stayed with us for the next two days to acquaint us with local areas and essential shopping. Khush was a person with a big heart who had been in touch with us since Divyansh's transplantation in Jerusalem in 2015. He often offered to help Sushil financially, which he always declined politely with thanks. Our relationship with him was distant, and we had never met each other till he came to receive us at the airport that day. Khush was a light-hearted, jovial and unassuming person, always willing to help without a fuss, a rare attribute to find amongst the Indian diaspora there. Every noble activity makes room for itself. Whatever Khush was doing for us, it just flowed naturally from him. Khush, in the short time spent with us, developed an excellent chemistry with Divyansh. Actually, his pleasing presence in the first two days laid a solid foundation to combat our tough days ahead. He left just a day before we were due to go to the hospital with a promise to come again to meet us.

Divyansh was advised by the treating doctor to first undergo a series of tests before a decision could be taken regarding his suitability for the trial treatment. To begin with, our experience of dealing with the people running and managing hospitals in USA was completely different from what we had at the Hadassah Hospital in Jerusalem. The profoundly humane element in the treatment we had witnessed in Jerusalem was somewhat lacking here. Even the Indian doctors who worked here were not forthcoming in helping and advising us informally. Well, that's a fact of life in USA, and we understood it in our early days.

All the tests reports came in the next three days, revealing that Divyansh was in complete remission. No malignant cells were found either in the CNS or in the bone marrow. This happened due to the doses of intrathecal Methotrexate by Dr Saikia before our travel to USA. Remission in medical parlance means malignant cells are not detectable in the patient's body. This didn't mean that the malignant cells would not come back. Since, in Divyansh's case, the treating doctor could not find the presence of the benchmark disease, the trial treatment was not approved. Trial treatments are normally sponsored by pharmaceutical companies, which generally approve such treatments in patients who report active diseased condition, so that after the trial treatment, they can compare the condition of the patients with the initial diseased condition to assess the potency and efficacy of the treatment. That's how their system works and Divyansh wasn't eligible for this. Sushil advised the doctor to let Divyansh remain without treatment for few days, hoping for the return of malignant cells. He would then become a suitable candidate for the trial treatment once he exhibited the benchmark diseased condition. The doctor was not enthused with this idea. He prescribed Divyansh a higher dose of intrathecal Methotrexate, apart from some other medicines which were tried on him in Jerusalem, which hadn't given him enduring benefit. The total stay for the prescribed treatment was going to be a little over a month. We had no choice but to accept the doctor's advice.

In hindsight, the doctor's blunder was going ahead with this treatment.

The treatment was started in the second week of April, and Divyansh had to be hospitalized for four days. Subsequent treatment was to be taken in day-care. Alongside his treatment, Divyansh began preparing for TOEFL and SAT, scheduled for late May and early June. This time, the side effects of the treatment were too painful and unmanageable. Yet, he tried his level best to manage his studies. There was no fear in his eyes about the treatment he was undergoing. He had profound self-belief in his karma. Treatment and studies—how could he stop writing blogs and poems alongside? Writing them became his novel way of reflection which would strengthen his life forces. They were not impediments. They were vital nutrients of blood which would infuse him with a fresh gush of energy to face and negotiate the challenges he faced.

Some of Sushil's college friends were residents of the city we were in. Suryakant Rajan, Shreevikas and Rajnish Chowdhary are names I must mention. They extended all possible help to make our stay comfortable. Rajnish Chowdhary, particularly, visited us regularly and often took us to his home outside the city for dinner. He was an attorney and had earned a good reputation in his profession. Apart from his work, he was actively involved in activities concerning the Indian diaspora there. His father too had been a cancer patient who had successfully recovered after the treatment. He knew the pain we were going through and I could make out the extent of empathy he had for us. He too, like many others, became Divyansh's admirer in the short time he spent with him.

Anshoo's wedding was on 22 April. It was our long-cherished wish to attend his wedding along with Divyansh. Divyansh, too, nurtured an intense desire to attend his wedding after missing Mridul's wedding earlier. It is difficult to control time and tides. What we can do is chart out ways through them. After abandoning the idea of attending his wedding because of the relapse and our travel to USA, Divyansh still attempted to brace the spirit of his wedding from long distance. To soak in the pleasure of Anshoo's wedding was still in his hands. But that needed him to get regular bytes from Anshoo and Mridul about various activities of the wedding. He wanted Anshoo to share the excitement he was going through, so that he could live it with him. Inexplicably, Divyansh was kept in the dark. Nothing of this sort came from them. This was too much for him to handle. Time is witness to the fact that he had faced the severest of challenges in his life with poise. He had made compromises with what was beyond his control, his relapse making him unavailable to be a part of this wedding. It was not a wedding of just any relative. This was one of his closest cousins and pals. He was completely deprived of the emotional feed from Anshoo and Mridul, which he really deserved. He made few attempts to contact them and take updates on the wedding, but the inputs he got were in complete disregard to their relationship. Maybe Anshoo and his parents thought it inappropriate to share their moments of happiness whilst we were going through our toughest times to pull back Divyansh from the brink of his life. But it was also a fact that we had given consent to them to go ahead with their wedding despite our extreme predicament. Divyansh could handle his physical and mental challenges stoutly, but when it came to bearing the pain of his wilful neglect by them, he couldn't. After all, he was only in his teens then. He still wanted to enjoy the wedding in his own way. Can't a person in pain and misery share and enjoy the happiness of others? Divyansh thought so. Sadly, they didn't. As for me, I was feeling equally let down. Anshoo himself was like another Divyansh for me. Didn't he owe it to send me his wedding photograph in the sherwani I had affectionately selected for him? Unknowingly, he didn't consider it fit to seek my motherly blessings as he stepped into his new life. This act of his shattered me.

One day, after we returned from the day-care centre, Divyansh cried inconsolably. I had never seen him cry like this before. We were quite upset thinking that it was some issues relating to the side effects of the medicine. After much consoling and cajoling, he spoke his mind about the emotional storm caused by their neglect and the feeling of being left out by them. Divyansh's level of commitment to them was unassailable. For the first time, the circumstances posed a question on the integrity of their relationship with Divyansh by their own conduct. That was the last time Divyansh was sad because of their indifference towards him. He moved on after that and never ever expressed his grief or annoyance with them. He was quite positive and jovial whenever he spoke to them. But the built-in trust of years had been dented. It was easier for Divyansh to make peace with himself because life had showered on him the virtues of wisdom and perseverance. But not a mother like me. I was a lesser mortal. It was too much for a mother to see the utter neglect of her son when he needed them the most in the toughest time of his life. A deep scar was etched in my heart.

That was when Divyansh wrote a poem 'Blood Is Thicker than Water'. Relationships tied with blood are those which unconditionally come out of their comfort zones to stand behind each other in trying times. The DNA of such relationships is metaphorically the vital electrolytes of the blood, which sustain them in good stead. The potency of such relationships for their eternal subsistence should not be blood-thinning external agents like aspirin, but this very vital electrolytic sinew. Some excerpts are as follows:

> Blood is thicker than water.
> But some are thinners like aspirin.

While vital electrolyte are few those,
Not sharing the same blood.

...

Aspirin, restrained by need,
Electrolytes, parched runs whenever,
The mental compass—disillusioned, giddy,
Will set charter in good stead,
The essential twins—
State of mind,
Peace of soul.

15

THE GRASS IS GREENER
ON THE OTHER SIDE

The treatment was progressing as planned. But this time, Divyansh faced too much difficulty. Yet he continued his preparation for SAT and TOEFL alongside, punctuated by the exposition of his thoughts on his literary canvas. Despite being his mother, who knew him the best, I was clueless as to how he had been able to manage both together. The sense of sovereignty which came to his life through all the turbulent phases in his past years had made him proficient enough to handle all these tasks together. As for treatment, I was not very sure if we were going in right direction. Sushil too was not satisfied with the line of treatment the doctor had prescribed. After all, he had been treating his son right under his care for the last eight years, and so, his gut feeling said different. Despite these difficulties and apprehensions, we tried to spend our time in harmony with our daily chores. We used to walk almost every morning, visit malls for occasional shopping, and sometimes, we ventured for dine-outs. Indulging in such acts flowed naturally from us, so we were able to maintain peace with the challenging times we were going through.

Since we were planning to get Divyansh admitted in a university in USA, we went to visit a prestigious local university. The kind of environment I saw there was tempting, forcing me to nurture a dream for Divyansh again. Divyansh easily sensed my feeling: What is actually seen on the other side is not always true. One should not disregard one's own possession in the dazzle of another's. Love and respect for one's own possession make it shine more than what we see on other side, and bring ever-lasting contentment. This was what he meant, I realized, in the poem he had written on 1 January that year. The poem was titled 'The Grass Is Greener on the Other Side'. Here is an excerpt:

> Bat off this desire with contentment,
> Respect and love are the moist drops,
> Greenery that paint,
> Onto all our possessions;
> Bringing a gleam greener,
> Than on the other side.

This poem was a timely reminder for me to value one's own possession.

To my great satisfaction, thanks to my parents, Ananya showed her remarkable persona while living without me for the first time. There was not a whisper of complaint from her to me to return early. Every time I called her, she said she was fine. Maybe time had realized a new whole in herself. And why not? Her journey, as Divyansh wrote in his poem, from Ayya to Bhaiya was yet to be completed. The time she spent in my absence provided her a perfect opportunity to give it a final touch.

As Divyansh proceeded towards the end of the treatment there, he began to experience discomforting side effects. It seemed to us that this could be because of higher doses of intrathecal Methotrexate. The doctor was the best judge to assess the efficacy of the treatment; however, we always presented to him all these symptoms in real time and took his advice. The personal touch of Dr Reuven Or was conspicuous by its absence here. We were to return to New Jersey on 13 May. The doctor suggested continuing the remaining part of the treatment in Mumbai. But whatever treatment Divyansh was undergoing, Sushil felt that sooner or later, malignancy would return. If that happened, we would certainly opt for the trial treatment. With this in mind, Sushil often told Divyansh that he needed to fight the battle one more time, perhaps, for the last time.

We returned to New Jersey to Ajay's home on 13 May. Divyansh and I were to stay there till the first week of June to finish SAT and TOEFL, after which we would fly to Mumbai. Sushil planned to return to Mumbai immediately. Ajay had earmarked a dedicated place in his house for Divyansh to study. He helped me coordinate with a local hospital to continue taking periodical treatment as prescribed. Divyansh had a homely atmosphere to relax in and study, after his protracted treatment and discomforting side effects in Texas. I, too, gradually adjusted to his family. Divyansh gelled well with Ajay's two daughters, Shreya and Shruti. Ajay genuinely looked invested in Divyansh and advised him all the time. He pictured a bright future if he continued his study and treatment in USA. Over time, the camaraderie between them grew so much that Divyansh often waited for him to return from work for lunch or dinner. Whenever Divyansh called him for anything, he was ready at his beck and call. I wondered at seeing Ajay's nobility and his growing fondness for Divyansh.

Sushil left for Mumbai on 15 May. Divyansh penned a poem after his father left for Mumbai to be with Ananya. When Sushil landed in Mumbai, Divyansh's poem was waiting in his inbox. Sushil opened the mail somewhere near the Sea Link, and couldn't stop his tears after reading it.

The hallmark of sibling unity is togetherness cemented through the common bond of their parents. With them, they play the game of life. Circumstances change and priorities too as the game progresses. The predicament of a parent sometime forces them to be either with the son or the daughter at a time to discharge their parental responsibilities. Yet, the brother-and-sister game continues—the game they play together and the game which time plays with them.

Who is this 'ball' in our lives?

The dynamics between these two siblings is metaphorically described through a ball representing their parents. It is also dedicated to their father who had to frequent travel between USA and Mumbai to take care of them in the best possible way. An excerpt is as follows:

So here we go, sister,
I have held the ball a long time,
Admiring it, tossing it vertically,
While your eager, yet patient eyes look on,
Curious for the next throw.

Hold on to the ball for me,
While I tie my shoe laces,
Adjust my cap, knocked off by the wind,
And steady my stance,
Shaken by fickle fate.

Since Sushil left for Mumbai, I tried my level best to adopt Ajay's home as mine. His house was a big one, but according to my own aesthetic sense, there wasn't much of an orderly system in place there. Most of them were late risers in the morning, except Ajay who had to get ready for his official duty by 8 a.m. We were always early risers and lived every moment of the morning solitude in all its niceties. Ajay's home was no different for us. Divyansh and I rose early in the morning and spent the morning in the living area which was an extension of the kitchen. Ajay also joined us and we enjoyed our morning tea together. That was when Divyansh and Ajay interacted a lot, which laid the foundation of their closeness and mutual admiration.

Divyansh, true to his humble nature and wisdom, had an excellent rapport with Ajay's daughters. His elder daughter Shreya was a promising student at Rutgers and was a reserved person. The younger one, Shruti, was a somewhat timid girl, who Divyansh used to teach subjects to when she approached him for help. Divyansh helped her in studies even though he was in discomfort and upset because of the medication. I gradually began guiding them in doing yogasana. I also actively involved myself in their household work and tried to bring some semblance of order to their kitchen.

To instil confidence in Divyansh in the education system there, Ajay took Divyansh to various seminars organized by The Institute of Electric and Electronic Engineers (IEEE) of which he was a key office bearer. He introduced Divyansh to the dignitaries on the dais and generally spoke to them about his brilliance and tenacity. Divyansh became a regular feature in the group photographs at the end of the programmes. All this led him to dream about a better life for him there.

Divyansh finished SAT and TOEFL in the first week of June, faring decently. Our return to Mumbai was booked for 12 June. The plan was to let Divyansh finish his second semester exams in Mumbai whilst undergoing treatment, and depending on his scores in SAT and TOEFL, a decision would be taken about our next visit to USA. From everything I heard from Ajay and others in USA, the earliest Divyansh could have gotten admission in any undergraduate programme would be spring semester beginning February 2018. He was too late for the fall semester, which would start in September 2017, but we still hoped to make it then. Ajay too tried his best to secure admission for Divyansh.

A week before our travel, Sushil called Ajay to discuss our return to Mumbai. Ajay had something else in his mind. He convinced Sushil that the idea of Divyansh's treatment and continuance of his studies in Mumbai was not at all a practical idea. It would ruin his future prospects in USA. Ajay promised his unstinting services on both counts for him: medical and academic.

He threw open his house for us and almost compelled Sushil to drop the idea of calling us back. He thought that if, by any chance, Divyansh got admission in the coming fall semester, it would be a futile exercise to go back to Mumbai at this stage.

The proposal that Ajay threw to us—we had never thought about it. So far we had stayed at his home under compelling circumstances. Hereafter, it would be too much for our dignity to continue to stay and also for his family to continue hosting us. We didn't know how long then. Sushil, on the other hand, knew from day one that Divyansh had no future in Mumbai. Apart from this, one of Divyansh's prescribed medicines was not available in India, and he had somehow got ready one reputed doctor to do this in Mumbai. Ajay's heaven-sent suggestion and his willingness to help Divyansh in whatever way possible changed our minds. We thought it was a matter of couple of months and in between Divyansh would have to go to Mumbai to finish his college second semester exams. When we asked Divyansh about it, he expressed his willingness to try his luck in USA.

So, the whole plan changed. The return tickets were cancelled. Was this for a purpose? Was this another dot the thread was attempting to join?

16

YOU SEE, I HAVE RENOUNCED FEAR

The people who matter to us and who leave a great legacy of good work and moral values are often forgotten after their deaths. It is expected that their souls should not only thrive in us, but also in our deeds as a mark of tribute to them.

Why can't we become the embodiment of those departed souls and spread the values inculcated by them for a better world?

With this thought in mind, Divyansh wrote a poem titled 'Dearly Departed' in memory of his late grandfather, after his return to Mumbai was shelved. He told me he had been thinking for a long while about writing on this theme, which he could now do with peace of mind. Here are some excerpts:

Dearly departed,
We were kept apart,
By time and tide,
Your love, your memory,
Breaks the dubious labyrinth,
Spun by fate.

...

You will forever thrive,
In conscience, in actions, in visage.
Respect and honour you will enjoy,
Thriving in the realm,
Bowed in your memory.

Sushil then came to New Jeresy to be with us for some time and to understand Divyansh's treatment plan in a local hospital and talk to the doctors. Ananya's birthday was on 17 June. That's why, in just five days, Divyansh threw back the proverbial 'ball' to Ananya to play with on her fifteenth birthday. A friend of Sushil's texted him when he reached Mumbai: 'Welcome to Mumbai. I know you are torn between two places.'

Divyansh's SAT and TOEFL scores, which came around third week of June, were fairly decent considering the circumstances he was in. He, with the help of Ajay, applied to various universities with a glimmer of hope that he might make the fall semester. In his statement of purpose, Divyansh, inter alia, highlighted his compelling circumstances to study in USA and his good academic record all through, despite the challenging situations posed by his formidable nemesis.

Towards the end of June, Divyansh and I returned to Mumbai to enable him to finish his college second semester exams. The admission in USA was still unconfirmed and, if at all it happened, there was a question mark about its timing: fall or spring semester. It was, therefore, thought advisable to secure what was in Divyansh's hand. While we had all approbation of Divyansh's prowess to manage everything whatever came his way, be it treatment, SAT and TOEFL or now the semester examination in Mumbai, I felt pity for him every time he struggled with his suffering to make new ways for himself. It seemed suffering to me, not to him. Suffering is the gap between expectations and performance. Divyansh, time and again, diminished the gap by raising the bar of his performance to reach as close to his expectations as possible. Therefore, in his own eyes, the suffering was always dwarfed by his determined actions.

While his exams were going on, he wrote another poem, his twenty-third, titled 'Tug of War'. The poem delineated his mental state while facing multiple challenges in his life. It also, in a way, portrayed my own mental condition in the face of troubles time

had posed to him so capriciously. Life, at any moment, is always a
tug of war, and one is being pulled on either side: past and future.
What is contested upon is our present. The shadow of the bad
spell cast by the past may be seen as trying to pull our present
to its side, but our belief should be in the other contestant, the
future, which would finally be the victor, pulling us from the
labyrinth of darkness. It should be our strong conviction that the
hostile present resulting from the past has only transient value.
The poem was so inspiring that it would be a great injustice if I
failed to quote whole of it. Here it goes:

Tugged taut and tense,
By belligerence, devoid of slackness;
I stand contested upon,
In the absent present.

On one side is Future,
Shining a promising bright,
Flexing muscles of certainty and hope,
Grunting a willing groan.

The Past presents itself,
Standing in equal measure,
Gathering strength to hold on,
Unwilling to relent.

Stretched to the last muscle,
Pumped with ambition,
A tickle of assurance every now and then,
Is the minute difference,
That makes the victor victorious.

The Future commands this minute difference,
As I drift in transience,
Watching the Other slowly lose,
[Its] vice—draining and disillusioning.

> I wait for what's imminent,
> Groaning in patience, silent.
> As Tense Time twists—
> From falling past,
> To the Future, rising afresh.

Divyansh's phrase 'Falling past to the future, rising afresh' showed a remarkable equanimity while facing challenges galore in his life! This poem made me see myself through my own eyes.

This poem was equally lived in letter and spirit by Ananya. When she met Divyansh and me after three months of abyss in her life, her expression was remarkably measured. She evoked a lot through her eyes, and only through her eyes—her craving for us, her worry about Divyansh and hope for our enduring family reunion. We acknowledged her intensity of emotion in the same way—through eyes only. As for Divyansh, it was as if he was seeing his own life through her verdant charm. Bhaiya was meeting her as Ayya. Without a doubt, she had been a silent collaborator with Divyansh in his battle for life for the past many years.

By mid-July, 2017, Divyansh and I returned to New Jersey to Ajay's home to continue his treatment and also to go all out to secure his admission in the fall semester, though Ajay often appeared circumspect about it.

When we returned this time, I found a little bit of uneasiness amongst Ajay's family members. Maybe they wondered how long they would have to host us. Perhaps they were right. We, on the other hand, were completely driven by our destiny. We often requested Ajay to look for a rented accommodation in the neighbourhood. But he always rejected the idea, emphatically saying that his house was ours and it would be absolutely inappropriate on his part to allow us to stay outside in the absence of Sushil, more so when he loved and cared for Divyansh so much. I was sandwiched between my moral duties—emotionally, I was driven by Ajay to stay with his family, but from a practical stand point, we should have stayed in a rented apartment. But one thing was sure; I did not feel the comfort now that I had enjoyed the last time. A feeling of unnerving helplessness gradually permeated into me.

In New Jersey, I regularly visited the hospital for Divyansh's treatment. Sushil was in Mumbai, so I took on the cudgel of his treatment. My initiation had begun in the Texas hospital, where I underwent a hands-on training to maintain the PICC line through which IV fluids were injected. It was a delicate task which only paramedics did in Jerusalem and India. The PICC line is normally maintained for a long time till the treatment lasts, so caregivers in US hospitals are advised to train themselves in its maintenance. Sushil and I both underwent this hands-on training. In a couple of sessions, I could perform to the satisfaction of the trainers. Though Sushil also grasped how to handle its maintenance, he often told me to do it as he felt I was more proficient in handling these affairs. When it comes to taking delicate care of children, a mother is the safest bet, he would often remark. Over time, Divyansh too preferred my tender touch for this job. Sushil had been handling Divyansh's personal care for the last eight years, where he did everything for him, including medical management. He never engaged anyone for Divyansh's medical care. He took it upon himself so assiduously that he would not be satisfied if others handled this. Divyansh felt for his father now. He was looking for a chance when he could free him from his ceaseless burden. After all, he was growing up and could empathize with him. Texas provided Divyansh and me this opportunity. My gradual initiation with hands-on training in PICC line maintenance was the first window Divyansh found to free Sushil from his day-to-day medical management to an extent. In hindsight, I felt it was Divyansh's deliberate ploy to prefer me for maintaining his PICC line to free his father from the onerous duty he had been performing for a long time. However, apart from this small task, Sushil handled all matters relating to his treatment in Texas personally. Even in our weekly meetings with the doctor, Sushil did most of the talking. In the initial days, I had a tough time understanding the heavily accented American English, which also forced me to take refuge under Sushil's leadership.

I began taking lead in helping Divyansh in his treatments and talking to the doctors, though I understood what they spoke only with great difficulty. Divyansh smartly used to intervene to save me from embarrassment whenever he thought it appropriate. He was also surely and consciously trying to take all aspects of his treatment in his own hands. One day, he told me as we left the hospital, 'Mummy, let me handle everything myself. Now I have to stay in USA. We don't know how long the treatment will go on. I should know to live with this and alongside, enjoy my life. Please go and get a cup of coffee for me to relax while the medication goes on.'

Life is meant to be lived and not to save for later days to enjoy. Pain or pleasure—one needs to live each moment to the fullest. That seemed to be the wisdom Divyansh practised through his tough days. I understand now that it was the gradual adjustment of his perception and attitude towards himself and his responsibilities towards his parents.

Ajay's boss, Dr Ulrich Rohde, was a scientist of international repute, holding no less than a 100 patents to his name. He heard about Divyansh and his heroic attitude. Dr Rohde, more than 85 years old then, invited all of us one day to his bungalow for a dinner. His wife, Ms Meta Rohde, was an equally affable person and a warm host. After the dinner, Dr Rohde talked to Divyansh at length and seemed swayed by his persona and his vision for a better world. That was possibly when Dr Rohde decided to write a recommendation letter for Divyansh, which could help him secure a college admission there. When I read his recommendation letter, I could only feel proud of Divyansh and bow in complete reverence to the humility of Dr Rohde. This was some of what Dr Rohde wrote:

> I am pleased to submit this letter in support of the above-referenced Mr Divyansh Atman Poddar for Undergraduate Admission in US University for Fall 2017 session. I have known Divyansh for more than five years. In my professional opinion, he is a uniquely well-deserved student for the undergraduate program at US University in Computer Engineering and Electronics Communication field. Divyansh is a well-disciplined, industrious student with a pleasant personality, energetic, compassionate and genuinely well-rounded. Through our interactions he has shown himself to be a hardworking school boy who is enthusiastic about new technology for the benefit of humanity.

Dr Rohde was perhaps another dot which the thread was joining.

We were now really hopeful that we would get calls for admission from the universities Divyansh had applied to.

It was Rakshabandhan Day. Divyansh was not with Ananya. But he was with two cousins this time—Shreya and Shruti. The flock of sisters that he would vow to protect on this day was going to increase in number. The celebration was performed on video chat through which Ananya from Mumbai could see Divyansh tying her rakhi and, also, the other two sisters doing the same to Divyansh. While Ananya was visibly satisfied with some semblance of celebration made possible by technology, she was palpably uncomfortable seeing her Ayya sharing her exclusive love with the other two. Divyansh had bought two exclusive gifts for Shreya and Shruti considering their tastes. He had done some research about their likes a day before and gone to the market to shop for those gifts. Gifts are mundane. But when given with some thought, they become priceless.

Ajay didn't have a sister. While the celebration of

Rakshabandhan was going on with all fervour, he spontaneously said to me, 'Bhabhi, I do not have a sister. Why don't you become my sister and tie a rakhi on my wrist?' His request was so sudden, I didn't think too much and just tied an extra rakhi from the tray on his wrist. He was very happy after that. He said that since he was now my brother, he would henceforth discharge all obligations of a brother towards his sister.

By the end of July, Divyansh, to our surprise, and Ajay's too, got calls from three universities for his admission. The first among them, the famous Drexel University of Philadelphia, offered him admission in his subject of choice, i.e., Computer Science. We were happy to get at least one offer for the fall semester we were vying for. The only and significant problem was that it was far from New Jersey, and considering Divyansh's medical condition and his need to take uninterrupted treatment in a local hospital in New Jersey, it would be impractical to take admission there. However, we bought time to confirm our assent to this university in case there were more such calls from other universities in the offing. Then, Divyansh got calls from two New Jersey universities: Drew University and Fairleigh Dickinson University (FDU). Divyansh had hit bull's-eye. We were so ecstatic that day that we did not hesitate to wake up Sushil by calling him at 2 o'clock IST that night. Now, we had to decide on the better option of the two.

Divyansh and I visited Drew University first, which was located in Madison, New Jersey. The registrar of the university had gone through Divyansh's CV, his SOP and the recommendation letter from Dr Ulrich Rohde. He was so impressed that he came to receive us at the gate and accompanied us through the campus visit. Drew was nicknamed 'The University in the Forest' because of its giant wooded campus. I was told that several motion pictures, TV productions and music videos have used this university as a filming location. Its academic buildings featured a mix of Greek and Gothic architecture. It was like a dream for me to imagine

Divyansh as a part of this grand college. And finally, the registrar not only confirmed admission in Computer Science in the fall semester but offered to enrol him directly in the second year, as Divyansh had already completed a year of his studies in college in Mumbai in the same subject. This would save a year of loss to him. The icing on the cake was the offer to Divyansh of a scholarship of 50 per cent of the college fees. Universities in USA rarely give scholarships for undergraduate programmes. Divyansh got that. But the most heartening thing for me was when the registrar told us that it would be a privilege for his university if a person like Divyansh studied in its college. I don't know how Divyansh took that comment, but for me, it was a moment of redemption for my son. It was all his auras, of which I considered myself a minuscule part.

Next stop was FDU after a couple of days. The campus of the university, a visual delight spread across both sides of a river, was just five miles away from Ajay's residence and very close to the hospital where Divyansh was taking treatment. The university offered him Electrical Engineering in the coming fall semester, which Ajay had suggested Divyansh should take up. After a few days, Divyansh got an email from the university confirming a 100 per cent scholarship for his studies, along with single room dorm. We had not applied for scholarship at either of the universities. At FDU, the entire quorum of the Scholarship Committee approved a 100 per cent scholarship considering Divyansh's meritocracy. At this stage, I was trying to connect Ajay's 1 January call this year advising us to consider Divyansh's studies in USA and this—the final stop at FDU just a few kilometres away from his home. We seemed to be driven by some mythical force.

Taking all aspects into consideration, Divyansh decided to join FDU.

Now, the next road block stared at us. Till now, Divyansh was on a tourist visa in USA. In order to secure a college admission to study in USA, he would have to return to Mumbai and apply for an F1 Visa at the US Consulate. The time left was too short to go to Mumbai, apply for the F1 Visa and wait for the interview call and the possibility of the Consulate office taking its own time to process the visa request. We were already in the first week of August when his admission for the fall semester was confirmed by FDU and was scheduled for 21 August. The admission in-charge for the international students of FDU was sceptical about Divyansh securing the F1 Visa in such a short time, considering his past experiences with other students. If he couldn't, then he would have to wait till the spring semester. Anyway, we took chance and flew back to Mumbai on 11 August. The visa application had already been made online two days before flying to Mumbai, with a request to consider it on an emergency basis. We were hoping against hope. Divyansh's visa interview was done on 13 August and the authorities sanctioned his visa request and wished him all the best with smiles. He got his F1 Visa with lightning speed in three days. Divyansh was very happy get it in time. Our joy knew no bounds to see the prospect of his dream of studying in USA finally coming to fruition.

Were all these lightning-fast occurrences leading Divyansh to join another dot?

Since a few days, Ananya had looked gloomy. She had realized that Divyansh would now live in USA, away from her, for his studies. Divyansh had been her constant support, both moral and material, as she grew. Of all of us, she was closest to him, and the only one she shared her feeling and problems with. She was going to miss the strong pillar of support which she had been leaning on so far. She knew that. However, her pensive thoughts did not reflect on her face. Divyansh had probably read that through the password he had to open her Pandora's box and unravel all that was going on in her mind at the conscious and subconscious levels. He discussed it with her privately and assuaged her anxiety by promising to video chat with her every day. She was surely going to miss her protector and guide in his physical absence. Before leaving, he cleaned his study table, book racks and drawers and put his belongings in order. He told Ananya to use his belongings whenever she wanted. In the evening, he took her to a nearby Starbucks café for a treat. I saw that Ananya always preferred to go out with Divyansh more than with us. He knew that too, and so he often took her out for some quick masti, as he would say.

We were packing to leave for USA. Sushil was going along with us and his plan was to stay there till Divyansh settled in the college. And then, a big alarm signal shook all of us. Just a day before our travel, Divyansh had the first stroke of the neurological storm brewing inside him. For a minute, all of a sudden, his speech became slurred and he could barely move his limbs. I was not home and Sushil was at office. Divyansh managed to call me and narrated this new development. I rushed to him. Sushil also came immediately. For two–three minutes, we didn't know how to react. It was impossible to contact the doctor who he saw in New Jersey. Doctors in USA do not share even their personal email ids, forget mobile numbers. There is a strict protocol to contact them there. We tried desperately to contact Dr Saikia but he didn't answer our call. Perhaps he was busy with his patients. The principled Dr Saikia consciously avoided taking calls from his patients and their caregivers. But he always responded to their emails or text messages as soon as he got the time. Theoretically, this practice can never be faulted. But emergency situations such as ours on that day can't be addressed through text messages. That would take time. I think in such situations, it is imperative for doctors to take calls from patients whose tough medical conditions they are aware of. It's a professional hazard for a doctor, but it can't be dispensed with. Having failed to reach him, we consciously avoided contacting other Mumbai-based doctors to avoid delay in travel to USA. Perforce, Sushil contacted our most reliable doctor,

Dr Reuven Or on his mobile, who instantly picked up his call and prescribed some oral medication for Divyansh immediately. The medicines he prescribed worked miraculously and he was fine in an hour. However, both Dr Or and we knew that it was short-term relief and it would surely return once he was off that magic pill. For some time, again Divyansh's prospect of studying in USA became a distant dream.

To our utmost relief, Divyansh didn't exhibit another attack before our departure to USA. We took this as a one-off episode and wanted to move on without thinking too much about it. The plan was to consult his doctor in New Jersey soon after reaching there and to take his advice.

I was also mindful of the fact that Divyansh was always subjected to the ferocious impact of time whenever he gained a foothold in either the personal or the academic front. This particular event seemed no different. I was shell-shocked. Divyansh, after recovering from this bout, told me pensively, 'Mummy, I feel cheated. I got my F1 Visa against all odds yesterday. And today, this new problem has cropped up. I feel someone is brutally pulling me back as I take a fresh stride.' I couldn't respond to this. However, we got busy preparing to travel. He, too, put a smile on his face, at the thought of a new life in USA.

You see, I have renounced fear,

And over optimism, and expectation.

I will move ahead from here,

With a numbness tempered by determination,

guts, patience,

And denial

('Catharsis')

17

THE UBER RIDE

We left for USA on 19 August.

Ajay was at the airport to receive us. He was happy to see that Divyansh was okay, as he was worried for him after the episode of neurological numbness a day before our travel. All through the drive home, he painted a bright future for Divyansh in USA and complimented him on getting his F1 Visa in record time.

The attending oncologist, Dr James Mac (pseudonym), after Divyansh's physical examination, commented that at this stage, he didn't require any intervention as he was fine then. However, he advised us to bring him forthwith if the symptoms of neurological numbness were repeated. The doctor was particularly pleased with Divyansh for having secured admission in FDU in record time and advised him to let loose his youthfulness in campus. We were relieved after consultation with the doctor, thus, ensuring no new stumbling block in Divyansh's college life in FDU.

The admission was granted the same day. We were asked to come the next day for the orientation programme. We were all there at 10 a.m. sharp. The big hall where we sat was full of students from various countries. Seeing Divyansh amongst them gave us a feeling of accomplishment. What a long way Divyansh had to travel to reach there and how he had done that: I was filled with intense thoughts, changing in multitudinous ways across the spectrum of past, present and future. The feeling of accomplishment was more profound with the way Divyansh made it to the fall semester against all odds. In less than six months, my perception about his life changed. In the month of March that year, Dr Saikia had advised us to allow him to live his life without any treatment and without any hope. In USA, a day before the admission, the consulting doctor too said the same thing though in a different perspective: to let him enjoy his life but with treatment and promising hope. The feeling of hopelessness had given way to hopefulness. *I will move ahead with denial.* Bravo, Divyansh, you made it today!

After the orientation we were led for the campus visit: the various departments, hostels, library, recreation centre, indoor basketball court and other things. I visualized Divyansh enjoying every bit of all this in the coming days as we moved from one place to the other. I noticed that day that Divyansh was trying to do everything on his own without our help. He stopped his father whenever he came forward to engage with him. After all, considering the medical condition he was in and the recent episode of neurological numbness, we couldn't have left him alone there.

The single room dorm Divyansh was allotted was a big one on the ground floor, with an attached toilet-cum-bathroom. A lush green carpet of grass across the window welcomed him, adding serenity to the ambience. How pleasurable was the shopping to set up his hostel room! The bed covers, pillows, stationery, toiletries, shoe-rack, rug, etc. It was particularly fascinating to buy a pair of coffee mugs with the letters D (Divyansh) and A (Atman) embossed on them. Each and every thing we bought felt like a fresh breeze in our lives. I set up his room with my own hands and arranged his clothes in the wardrobe to ensure that the tender touch of my motherhood remained there with him without me. The campus security officer knew about Divyansh and came to see him at his dorm and advised him to call him if he needed anything. Personally, I was not happy with the single room Divyansh was to live in. I feared that would leave him in perpetual loneliness. I wanted him to enjoy life with a roommate and indulge in all the youth-centric activities he had missed so far. But considering the possibility of catching infections from a room partner, the college authorities were right in allotting him a single occupancy dorm.

As a part of the orientation, the college had organized a group excursion to New York City. I was a bit reluctant to allow him on this excursion, considering his recent episode. I then remembered the doctor's advice to let him enjoy his youth. Divyansh went on that trip. He sent a number of pictures to us while on tour. He bought souvenirs for his father and Ajay when he returned from the trip, which had them enraptured.

Sushil was to return to Mumbai on 28 August. He had spent almost 12 years of his life in hostels. Divyansh was to spend the first night of his life in a hostel on 27 August. Sushil stayed with him in the hostel, though Divyansh had only reluctantly agreed to the idea. That night Sushil shared various anecdotes of his hostel life with him and generally tried to keep him upbeat about the exciting days ahead. The next day morning, before leaving to attend classes, Divyansh ordered an Uber for Sushil to take him to Ajay's home. Whilst leaving, Sushil gave him a tight hug with moist eyes as he was to leave for Mumbai the same evening. Sushil couldn't hold his emotions and was choked as he stepped into the cab thinking that Divyansh would now have to manage everything on his own, along with the baggage of medical problems. He was more concerned due to the recent episode of neuro-seizure. He was being pulled on three sides: by Divyansh, Ananya and his job. So far, he had been managing his responsibilities towards all three with tremendous astuteness. He actually wanted to stay more with Divyansh before his return to Mumbai but had to decide against it.

Divyansh called Sushil that evening as he was leaving for the airport. But as Sushil talked to him, he abruptly disconnected the phone. We all grew tense, wondering what had happened to him. We couldn't figure out what led him to behave like this. Eventually, he called again and told Sushil that he was unable to hold back his tears while talking to him, thinking how emotionally difficult it was going to be for him to go on without Sushil's physical presence. Sushil had been with Divyansh like his shadow since 2009 when he was diagnosed with leukaemia. So, Divyansh felt for the first time that from now on, he would have to manage without his solid support system. The only saving grace was that I would continue to stay with him in New Jersey, though not with him in the hostel.

Divyansh gradually adjusted to the college campus. He regularly attended classes, and in between, visited the hospital for his periodic check-ups and treatment. Classes, treatment and weekends at Ajay's home became the order of his days. In a short time, he established his mark of academic excellence and affable personality amongst both the teaching fraternity and students. He was one of the top scorers in various internal exams. The teachers were particularly appreciative of the way he stout-heartedly excelled in multiple faculties, against the physical limitations posed by his illness.

Though I wanted Divyansh to spend most of his time in the campus for his smooth adjustment, Ajay always encouraged him to come home to stay with him. More often than not, he would drive to his hostel after office hours and bring him back home. Divyansh too used to enjoy these off-campus occasions. Divyansh was with me in New Jersey, and Sushil was with Ananya and attending to his office duties in Mumbai. Our lives seemed somewhat on track, though we were mindfully walking on the edge.

In the second week of August, Ajay had to go for a business trip to Italy along with his family. It was a tough ask for me to live in his big bungalow alone while Divyansh stayed at the hostel. It was Ajay's very presence that gave me the psychological boost to face challenging situations there. I was very apprehensive about dealing with such situations in his absence. What would happen if Divyansh again had a neuro-seizure? How would I manage him alone? All these negatives thoughts flooded my mind.

It seemed the demon was waiting to hit us at an opportune time. Just the day after Ajay's departure to Italy, Divyansh called me from the dining room of the campus, managing to just say that he was not able to lift his hand. With great difficulty, he had managed to grab his mobile and call me. His speech sounded slurred. I was completely shaken, wondering what to do. There was no one around to help me. I called Sushil in Mumbai, who then called Divyansh to book an Uber and come to Ajay's home address. A determined Divyansh somehow managed to call Uber and reached Ajay's home. By that time, he felt a little better. In such situations, Ajay had often told me that one should immediately rush to the ER (emergency room) of a hospital. At that time, I didn't even know the meaning of ER. On Ajay's advice from Italy, Divyansh somehow dialled 911 to take him to the ER of the hospital he was taking treatment from. They immediately came and took us to the hospital.

It was tough for me to manage everything on my own in the hospital. I had never done that before. Sushil was not around and I missed him and felt like crying. But there was only me now to take care of Divyansh. I somehow regained my composure, evoked the motherhood that Divyansh eternally envisaged in me and began dealing with hospital issues. For the first time, I came out of the shadows of Sushil and Divyansh, directly talking to the doctors and nurses. It was awful for me talking to them and responding to their accented English. The faster one throws oneself in deep waters without helping hands, the sooner one learns the art of swimming. Crutches help you walk, but many a time, it stops you from realizing your true potential. That day, I was without any crutch. I was able to stretch myself beyond my own limitations. A gradual realization seeped through me that I was stepping into Sushil's shoes now to do what he would have done had he been with us then.

An MRI of the brain revealed some deformity. The treating doctor, Dr James Mac, against the opinion of the neuro-oncologist, Dr Sam Lerman (pseudonym), advised us that there was no need for any intervention by way of brain biopsy at this stage. In hindsight, this was a blunder.

We were discharged from the hospital on the third day. To my astonishment, Divyansh said he would go straight to the college from there to attend his classes. I was dumbfounded at his decision as I felt he needed rest after his hospital stay. He seemed to be racing against time and so went all out to do as much as possible, despite the severe constraints he was going through.

In a few days, Ajay and his family returned. As usual, Ajay drove to Divyansh's hostel to bring him to his home. That day, Divyansh went to the hospital via Uber to collect his medicines. He wrote a short piece on his blog wall about his experience with the Uber driver that day. It was so poignantly written, it moved me to tears. 'The Uber Ride' goes like this:

The Uber pulled into the driveway.
'You undergoing treatment in that cancer centre?'
'Yes, came to pick a prescription up,' came the tentative reply.
'You go man! Stay strong! Lost my ma to it, dad undergoing treatment. What's your age?'
'20?'
As the car pulled over at the destination, 'All the best man! I'll pray for you! You so young! 2–3 years down, and you'll be well settled into a married life!'
'Thanks man! Give my best to your dad!'
The smiles said farewell.

The Uber driver gave more than a ride. He got more than just the fare.

The student got more than a ride. A memory to cherish for days to come.

On returning from Italy, Ajay insisted that Divyansh should stay with him at home, considering his recent seizure. I did not want this. I wanted him to live a new life in the campus which he couldn't earlier. His dorm was hardly a 15-minute drive from Ajay's home, so if anything happened, we could be there in no time. I wanted him to keep challenging his comfort zones. Staying at Ajay's home was the easiest option. There was another reason I wanted Divyansh to stay in the dorm. Our prolonged stay at Ajay's home had generated some unwelcoming responses from his family members. Though never direct, I sensed their subtle presence. It unnerved me. I felt awkward to cook the kind of food I would have liked to feed Divyansh. The negativity created was sensed by Divyansh too. So he too avoided staying at Ajay's home, despite Ajay's best efforts. At the end of the day, which mother would not want to keep her son close to her in the situation Divyansh was in, more so when Sushil was not with us? For my decision, I was always subjected to Ajay's ridicule. Sushil, whenever he called from Mumbai, often requested Ajay to look for a rented accommodation nearby, which he kept avoiding.

One day, I was so pissed off with the annoying negativity that kept hurting my self-respect that I emphatically requested Ajay to look for an independent flat around Divyansh's college campus. I felt equally bad to see Ajay suffer because of us. He listened to me intently but told me that since he was now my brother, there was no question of me staying outside. I was at the receiving end of his well-intentioned moral crisis. All these factors only had me firmly insist that Divyansh stay in his dorm, barring his occasional visits on weekends. Sushil was soon expected to come, and we would then take a decision to shift our place of stay.

Divyansh gradually cemented his place on campus. Apart from his studies, he attended seminars and also joined yoga classes, which he attended after college hours. Alongside the college curriculum, he joined a course to learn a computer language at New Jersey Institute of Technology every Saturday. It was astounding for me to see him do so many things at the same time that, at times, it unsettled me. He seemed to be in complete denial of his medical condition and was racing against time to grab as much of his share of accomplishments as possible. He had accepted his life in whatever way it was offered to him. But time was not in sync with his indomitable spirit. I often visited his dorm in the evenings after his classes and spent some time with him. I would find him alone in his room. He avoided going out. I coaxed him to go out and spend some quality time with his friends. He never said anything. Something was brewing in his mind that I couldn't fathom. Perhaps he was getting some hints as to where he was heading, which we were not.

In early October, he got an opportunity to fulfil one more dream in his life: visit the UN office in New York when the college organized a trip for willing students to visit it. Divyansh in the past had participated in a MUN in Mumbai where he had represented Israel for making deliberations. Now, it was time for him to see and experience the UN General Assembly Hall live. His photo in a black suit, silver-grey shirt and matching printed tie clicked in the Assembly Hall showed how proud he was for having been able to make it there. He looked so complete in the selfie he had sent to his father that Sushil texted him, 'Your transformation is heavenly. Expect to get rid of your cap soon. I am dying to see that day in your life. Love you loads.'

The Chhath festival was fast approaching. How could I perform the rituals in USA at Ajay's home? As my stay there was prolonged for reasons beyond my control, this question loomed in my mind. The celebration of this festival required elaborate preparations and practice. Apart from the constraints of managing resources for this festival in New Jersey, there was the issue of the unfavourable atmosphere at Ajay's home which discouraged me from celebrating this festival. I didn't want to overburden them. Considering the impracticality of doing this from Ajay's home, Sushil advised me to drop the idea this time. I was cognizant of the fact that I had begun keeping a fast for this festival only for Divyansh's well-being. How could I drop this when he needed the fruit of my penance the most at that point in time? I also discerned from Divyansh's body language that he wanted me to celebrate the festival. By that time, I remained the only person in whom he could repose his unflinching faith, whose karma could supposedly pull him out of the difficult time he was in. When medicine doesn't work, prayer does. With this thought in mind and keeping at bay all discouraging factors, I decided to go ahead and observe Chhath. To be fair to Ajay, he managed all the necessary resources for my fasting and worship.

Divyansh accompanied me all through the rituals of this festival, just to make a point subconsciously that he, too, was doing the penance along with me and giving me moral, emotional and physical support. But, by then, Divyansh had begun to show early signs of his weakening physical flexibility due to neurological disturbances. Despite that, he supported me through the rituals. Ajay too stood rock-solid behind me. Time compelled me to celebrate this festival on alien soil. I had never thought about it. As I paid my obeisance to the Sun God, I prayed to him to shower his eternal blessings for a healthy life of my son. I must confess something was amiss in me, which did not let me feel spiritually content through the celebrations. But at the end of the day, I had some semblance of satisfaction of making it against all the odds. Along with Divyansh, I too was put to test by the same divinity whose intervention I beseeched for Divyansh's well-being. In our lore, observing the rigorous Chhath fast is considered the toughest. With Divyansh by my side and in my mind, this was no longer tough for me.

After Chhath, Sushil shared some good news with us. He had been promoted in the department he was working in, which was long overdue. He was actually waiting for this order before he planned his next visit to us. He thought he would take on the new charge after his promotion and then a long leave to be with us for Divyansh's treatment. I remember how happy Divyansh was when Sushil broke this news to him. He teasingly texted him, 'Congrats Papa, so, now you have become Commissioner. Proud of you.'

Sushil flight to New Jersey was booked for 18 November.

❦

18

PLUCKING THE STRINGS OF EMOTIONS

Man thrives, oddly enough, only in the presence of a challenging environment.

—L. Ron Hubbard

Divyansh steadily attempted to conquer challenges. His challenges kept him energized. They kept him alive. He was never satisfied whatever he was doing. He strived hard to be better. In the words of George Bernard Shaw, satisfaction was death for him.

The frequency of his neuro-seizures was increasing. We were worried and couldn't figure out what was happening to him. In our visits to the doctor, he didn't say anything that warranted immediate intervention. He only said it was the side effect of the drugs. We were sure that we hadn't missed anything from our end. We reported to the doctor the moment the seizures occurred. If at all anyone was missing in during the assessment of Divyansh's deteriorating medical condition, it was perhaps the doctor himself, which became clearer in the coming days. There were days I used to go to his dorm, stay with him during the day, accompany him to his classes and wait for them to get over.

One day, while waiting for Divyansh in the dorm to come back from classes, I got a call from him saying he had fallen down and was not able to move his limbs. I immediately rushed to the lecture hall where I found him sitting on a bench outside the hall. He smiled at me when I reached there. I was panic-stricken. He was not. After recovering from the bout, he went to the library to finish his work while I waited outside. He was definitely becoming neurologically poorer, with frequent numbness in his limbs causing him to fall. He was undeterred despite this. Even in this precarious condition, he sat for the internal examination and scored one of the highest marks in the class. Sitting at a distance outside his class, I could see how difficult it was for him to even keep his eyes open during lectures. In between, he raised his hands to ask questions too.

Divyansh's strongest companion through all his struggles was his mental strength, which unfailingly steered him through challenging times, no matter how difficult they were. It was still on display to me, though mentally, he was becoming slower and slower. Yet, he outshone other students in his class, to the amazement of the teachers. He craved study. His soul was holding his tired brain in its lap, debilitated by leukaemia and the side effects of the drugs, pushing him to study as much as he could. Time, in the face of ceaseless challenges to the resilient Divyansh through the past many years, could not take it anymore. It played an unholy game with him. In cowardly fashion, it hit his strongest ally: his sturdy mind. Time mischievously attempted to attack him from the rear while he slumbered. Divyansh was completely oblivious to what was happening in his brain. Yet, he was giving Time a tough fight. He was going down, but was still not out. All the while, he remembered his father's comment that he had to fight one more battle, probably for the last time. Sushil's remark was made in the context of his apprehension of the return of leukaemia in his brain, considering the ad-hoc treatment given to him in Texas. If that happened, then he wanted to put him in the trial treatment for a long-term solution.

Considering his physical restrictors and his anxiety about his studies, Divyansh wrote Ajay a mail on 10 November:

Dear Fufaji,

I am at a critical juncture of my semester. Booking subjects for next semester is going to take place in the coming weeks. Assignments are due, some are overdue. I am having difficulty in one subject. It is at this point where I have taken ill. I am unable to walk properly by myself. This has restricted me to bed rest, and missing out on college. If I am not in college, how will I look into these matters? Please help me. And copy the same to my chart, so that doctor understands my plight.

Ajay tried to help Divyansh on all counts, but he too was helpless about his deteriorating physical condition.

Sushil reached New Jersey on the morning of 19 November to be with his soulmates: Divyansh and me. Divyansh smiled when he saw him but nothing more than that. Sushil gave him a tight hug. He craved for something more from him as they were meeting after over two months. But something was amiss with Divyansh. He suspected some major problem in him. Hoping it would not be the worst, we took an appointment with the doctor for the next day. That night, Divyansh had difficult sleep. He remained awake till 1 a.m. despite his best efforts to sleep. We tried hard to make him sleep but in vain. I was transported in my trance to the days when Divyansh picked up playing the guitar with his passion for music.

Divyansh's medical treatment after the first relapse was very tedious and exhausting. The treatment protocol was sacrosanct and had to be followed scrupulously. He had to go twice a week to the day-care centre for the treatment and then grapple with its side effects and mood swings. Managing mood swings well was at his command.

In early 2013, he picked up string instruments—first, acoustic and later, bass guitar—to resonate with his soul. Slowly and steadily, the musical strings began to help him assimilate with the rhythm and melody of his life force. I had heard people saying music can lift the sagging spirit. It takes you to a different level. I saw this happen with Divyansh.

One day, Divyansh expressed a desire for some CDs of string-instrumental music. After work, Sushil went to the iconic Rhythm House at Kala Ghoda. He was struggling to select one which he thought Divyansh would like.

He politely asked a store boy to suggest to him the latest albums of string instruments. The store boy in bright red T-shirt guided him to a shelf and picked up *Plucked* and said, 'Sir, this is the latest from Niladri Kumar. He plays the zitar. You will like it. It is my personal favourite and hopefully will be yours too.'

Sushil had never heard the name of this instrument. He initially avoided asking the store boy what the zitar was to mask his lack of knowledge.

'Will it be to Divyansh's liking? Can *Plucked* really pluck Divyansh from his sombre mood?' A feeble voice came from within. Shedding his embarrassment, Sushil asked the store boy apologetically to explain what the zitar was, since it was new to his understanding. The store boy explained simply in layman terms that the zitar was an electric sitar.

With new knowledge of this instrument, he respected the recommendation of the boy and bought that CD. When Sushil handed the CD to Divyansh, he only wished the musical notes of this five-stringed instrument stood as a torch bearer of hope and fuelled him with energy to tread the roads ahead.

We played the tracks. The very first title track tore our hearts. We listened to the album together umpteen times. We would figure out the central theme of various tracks and try to imagine what must have gone on in the mind of the musician before composing the tracks.

The monsoons of 2014 had set in. It was raining incessantly in Mumbai. Sushil and Divyansh had just returned from the day-care centre. His college was closed for the next five days on account of a long weekend. Divyansh, seated in the balcony, read the *Mumbai Mirror*. He told Sushil that there was going to be a concert of Niladri Kumar at Liberty, Church Gate. Not sure if his wish would be fulfilled, he asked him tentatively, 'Is it possible we can watch the show together?'

Sushil didn't want to say no. Saying yes was a risky proposition as Divyansh had the propensity to catch infections in crowded places. However, Sushil said yes, with a caveat of approval from the treating doctor first. He didn't want to disappoint him. He also knew that if he had asked permission of the doctor, he would have been advised to avoid large gatherings. Sushil played a small trick and re-phrased the question. 'I intend to take Divyansh to a concert. What precautions do I need to exercise?' Sushil asked the doctor on the phone. With no option to say yes or no, the doctor advised him to avoid visibly sick people in the crowd. He didn't want to deprive Divyansh of his musical experience. Right from the beginning of the treatment, he had decided that the treatment and the kind of life he wished should go hand in hand. And that was how he had decided to live his life with his nemesis, which we accepted and admired.

It was 28 July 2014 at Liberty. Divyansh and Sushil reached in time, enjoying the melody and rhythm of raindrops along the way. The concert was superb. Niladri enthralled Divyansh. Sushil could see his upbeat mood when he played the track 'Plucked'.

Divyansh was a young man of few words. But when it came to writing, he poured his heart into it. The day after the show, he texted Sushil:

Papa, I thank you infinitely for taking me to the show yesterday. It was just the perfect retreat for my otherwise monotonous life. *Itna mazaa aaya* [I had a lot of fun]. I really felt a great sense of contentment, relief and bliss. It was an experience unmatched by the many materialistic things we do to feed our cravings. I feel so refreshed today that it is hard to describe. Thanks again.

Sometimes even a small act gives so much happiness that is hard to describe. As a father, Sushil felt this was one of those small things which lingers in his mind even today.

A couple of years later, Divyansh wrote on Niladri's Facebook wall:

Hello Sir,

I had heard your album *Plucked* a couple of years back. As the name suggests, it really 'plucks' the strings of the emotions and consciousness. Beautiful melodies and rhythms. Since then, [I] have been following your work, and have even attended two of your concerts. And both the experiences were a goosebump-inducing journey through tranquillity. You have a new fan in me, Sir. Will keep following your work.

With regards,

Divyansh Atman

And Niladri acknowledged his post.

Something came to our minds when we found Divyansh was not being able to sleep. The bluetooth speaker was always a part of our travel kit. Sushil instantly paired his phone with the bluetooth speaker and played 'Plucked', the strings of the zitar, thinking it might work. That night we witnessed the power of music. One by one, the tracks played: 'Plucked', 'Together', 'Touch the Sky', 'Prayers', 'Rivers', 'Right Meets Left'... Divyansh, with the soothing reverberation of strings, found his sleep. Like before, this time too, *Plucked* plucked him from his misery and transported him to the infinite tranquillity of sleep. It was a revelation to me. A person who, because of poor medical conditions, had almost failed to connect with his beloved father who he used to idolize, could do so with the music he listened to. All night long, Sushil played the same tracks on repeat mode. Divyansh didn't wake up from sleep till late in the morning. *Plucked* seemed to have plucked the strings of his emotions and consciousness. He was still inseparable from the strings he used to play and listen to. And why not? A child, right from his pre-natal stage, develops a sense of music when his mind is tuned to the rhythm of his mother's heartbeat.

Considering Divyansh's deteriorating neurological condition, Sushil suspected the return of malignant cells in his CNS. But he couldn't understand why he was in such a poor condition. The CNS relapses had happened in past too, many times. But he was never in such a poor physical condition. Over the last eight years, Sushil had almost become a doctor, able to read any changes happening in Divyansh at the very first instance of its appearance, and would then act fast. Here, too, though he had not been with us for the last two months, he was in constant touch with the doctor and would talk to him via video chat whenever we visited him. With or without him, we did what we could have done the best. There were no lapses from our side in missing any vital signs for timely intervention. In fact, the treating doctor got irritated with our frequent visits.

Divyansh was admitted to the hospital under the care of Dr Sam Lerman, the neuro-oncologist, on 21 November. No matter his physical and mental cognition at that time, Divyansh could only talk about his studies and upcoming exams at FDU. A series of MRIs showed the presence of lesions in the brain. However, a CSF test revealed that there were no malignant cells in the nervous system. The doctors were baffled by the nature of lesions in the brain which showed up in the MRI scan. The only way to find out was through a delicate and risky procedure of brain biopsy which the doctor had been avoiding for so long. As the days progressed, Divyansh was increasingly becoming neurologically weak. A time came when he could hardly swallow. It was difficult for him to sleep and he would continuously moan all night. I couldn't figure out what was happening to him. His moaning would stop when I touched him. He still was able to relate to the tender motherly touch. Sushil and I stayed with him in the hospital 24X7. We were shell-shocked, completely clueless about what would happen the next moment. The brain biopsy was planned for 28 November.

The treating oncologist Dr James Mac came in on the morning of 25 November to see Divyansh. Even he looked clueless after examining him. I had become so nervous that after the consultation, I held his hand and beseeched him, 'Doctor, please save my son. He deserves to see this world more.' The doctor empathized with me but said that his condition looked tough to manage. He observed that if it was a case of return of the malignant cells, he could possibly manage with the same trial treatment for which we had come to USA. However, before leaving, he roped in one noble social worker, Susan, for our emotional support and counselling.

Susan was a social worker attached to the hospital where Divyansh was being treated. The medical social workers lead support group discussions, provide individual counselling to patients and their caregivers and provide other health services. Susan, an old noble person, possibly in her 60s then, came to meet us the very next day. She was tall, fair-complexioned and possessed excellent communication skills. She spoke with remarkable poise and when she listened, I felt like speaking on and on to her. All through, her presence and her soothing smile helped me open my heart to her. She evoked unfathomable spirituality through her persona where I took refuge to get some mental solace.

Susan wanted to know about us, more particularly, about Divyansh. We talked at length. Sushil described to her Divyansh's heroic journey. She listened to him intently. She must see a lot of patients and their caregivers daily, but the way she engaged herself with us that day, it seemed like we were the first and last people she was working with. Such was the magnitude of her engagement. When Sushil finished talking, I took over from him. For me, the saddest plight was to see someone (Susan) look at my son in a distressed condition. He was not in good shape. I had given birth to Divyansh. When guests visited our home in his growing years as a kid, I took pride in dressing him up well and making him look presentable. I was going through the same motions when Susan came to visit us. Divyansh was not what she was seeing. I couldn't make my son as presentable then as I would have liked. The only way to do that was through my reflections to her about the real Divyansh, his resolute life, his unflinching faith in karma, his nobility and his literary and musical sojourn. I showed her Divyansh's photos and videos in my mobile gallery, made her read his poems and blog articles. I saw her gleaming eyes as she began to know Divyansh more. I garnered motherly satisfaction; I had now made my son captivating to her. Divyansh was worthy of it. It was my karma to bring forth his karma to others.

Susan, in the time she spent with me that day, read Divyansh's poem 'Here We Go Again' and liked it immensely. She was so moved that she couldn't resist commenting and wondering how a young boy of his age could think and write like that. She felt the poem needed to be read by one and all, especially those who were in difficult situations. After a long meeting, she bade us goodbye with a promise to visit again in the next few days. Before leaving, she shared her personal mobile number and email ID, saying we could reach out to her anytime.

19

TUG OF WAR

Divyansh was being wheeled to the OT Room for the brain biopsy. Sushil caressed his head, kissed him and wished him good luck. While he was in the OT, undergoing the procedure of extraction of tissues from a delicate part of the brain, Sushil speculated on various outcomes. As the doctor said, the tissue examination could either show malignancy or any infection: viral, bacterial or fungal. We felt that in all these scenarios, Divyansh was treatable. After a long wait, the doctor came out of the OT and called our names. The doctor told us in a relaxed manner that the first glance at the tissue extracted didn't suggest malignancy. The only outcome left to be diagnosed was the nature of infection, the result of which would be made available in the next two days. Scared at the prospect of the diagnosis going towards the old issues of malignancy, we were quite relieved to hear this. We felt that any infection could be taken care of.

Sushil was in regular touch with Dr Reuven Or. After understanding Divyansh's latest symptoms, he had mailed him even before the biopsy result came, suspecting post chemo-radiotherapy necrotizing encephalitis. In the event this was the final diagnosis, he suggested treatment by hyperbaric oxygen chamber.

The next few days were very traumatic. Divyansh's condition was fast deteriorating. Even two days after the tissue analysis, the doctor could not diagnose the nature of the lesions in his brain.

And until a final diagnosis was made, they could not prescribe any viable treatment protocol for Divyansh. Any wrong treatment could worsen his condition rather than help his cause. Having failed to figure out the nature of cells of the lesions, they finally sent the tissue sample to a well-known hospital in New York for analysis.

Divyansh had begun to aspirate his saliva into his lungs because of poor swallowing caused by impaired functioning of the brain. It was 2 December, our wedding anniversary. Sushil had bought a small bouquet from a gift store of the hospital we were in. His eyes were moist while he gave it to me. Our wedding anniversary didn't mean anything to us that day. The flowers never looked so pale before. We both knew. Sushil was unsuccessfully trying to look normal to me. Divyansh's oxygen saturation was fast dropping because of the aspiration of saliva into his lungs. The doctors and nursing staff tried hard to manage from the general ward we were in, but didn't succeed. They finally shifted him to the ICU by late evening for better care. We were shocked when he was being shifted to the ICU. Was the worst coming to us now?

By late night, his oxygen saturation could not be sustained at the desired level despite external oxygen sources. Seeing no alternative working, they decided to intubate him and put him on life support. Divyansh, on a ventilator? At such a young age? We became vegetative for some time. My neurological system stopped giving any stimuli to produce physical or emotional reactions. There was no one around except Sushil and I. Ajay was expected any time. We were absolutely blank as the nursing staff prepared to put Divyansh on ventilator. While he was sinking, I too was sinking. Sushil was trying to manage both of us, the mother and her son while they were sinking together. It looked like I would lose him in the next few hours. The life support, after a few hours, relieved Divyansh from the constant thumping of his chest caused by poor oxygen levels. He was transported into an abyss of deep slumber.

On 5 December 2017, the final diagnosis based on tissue analysis done by the hospital in New York arrived. Divyansh was suffering from leukoencephalopathy, which is nothing but necrotizing encephalitis as suspected by Dr Reuven Or. Leukoencephalopathy in the brain happens because of extreme toxicity caused by intrathecal Methotrexate, which results in the formation of lesions in the brain and starts killing brain cells. When Dr Sam Lerman came in the evening to discuss the biopsy results, he dropped a bombshell on us. He commented that the leukoencephalopathy had caused irreversible damage to the brain and the condition was only going to get worse in the next few days. He said there was no treatment for his medical condition except administering intravenous steroids to reduce the swelling in the brain. According to him, there were hardly hundred such cases reported worldwide so far and there was not much research done yet to devise effective treatment protocol for this medical condition. Another bombshell he dropped before leaving the ICU room was when he said, 'Don't expect he will survive for more than two months.' These discussions happened with Sushil, in my absence. Sushil, though extremely petrified with the line of Divyansh's survival drawn by the doctor, went on to ask him about the prospect of treatment by hyperbaric oxygen chamber as advised by Dr Reuven Or. The doctor didn't agree to his advice for the simple reason that Divyansh was not in senses to monitor and regulate oxygen flow inside the chamber. Besides, he also said that this treatment for leukoencephalopathy was not approved by FDA in USA. The doctor left the ICU in a huff after pronouncing these brutal sentences.

But why did Divyansh reach the stage of leukoencephalopathy? If this was the cause of his neuro-seizures that we had been reporting to Dr James Mac for the last three months, why didn't he act fast to diagnose the true nature of lesions? Why did the doctor wait so long, allowing irreversible damage to the brain? If treatment by hyperbaric oxygen chamber was a possibility, it could have been taken when Divyansh was cognitively active if the diagnosis had been made in time. Or did Dr James not have the experience of dealing with such rare medical conditions? All these questions plagued our minds. We suspected a medical lapse, negligence or error of judgement by the treating doctors which became clearer to us as the days progressed.

The next day, Susan came to the ICU looking for Divyansh's room. She found us standing outside his room discussing Divyansh's update with the ICU in-charge Dr Ching (pseudonym), a doctor of Chinese origin but a citizen of USA. She held a paper as she wished us good morning. When we had finished talking to the doctor, she expressed her deep concern on Divyansh's deteriorating medical condition. Then, she gave me the paper she was holding in her hand, to read. It was his poem 'Here We Go Again'. She had taken a printout of Divyansh's poem and wished to paste it in the ICU rooms of the patients. She said that when she had gone back home after meeting us last night, she read the poem again and was deeply moved by the underlying thought espoused through the poem. She felt that the poem was so empowering that all patients and their caregivers should read it. Susan was invoking us to come to terms with our pain with a device crafted by Divyansh—his poem. Taking my permission, she pasted the poem in the ICU rooms. In the next few days, the poem became a rage there and a talking point in the hospital. Doctors dropped by to Divyansh's room just to see him physically, the poet of 'Here We Go Again'. After reading Divyansh's poem, the nurses began feeling for him. The kind of pain I saw in them was as if they felt for their son or brother. When they came to his room, their eyes would invariably turn moist. One young nurse of Divyansh's age or just a little older to him devoted herself to taking such deep care of him as she would her own brother. Divyansh lay quiet. He was like any other patient the nurses served. It was his empowering poem that touched their souls. Through his poem, he glowed ethereally, so profoundly that he carved a permanent place in their hearts.

Nurses took copies of the poem with our permission, saying that this poem needed to be read again and again by one and all. Obviously, in the ICU, Divyansh had become a talking point and began commanding huge respect; all this whilst he was in deep sleep on life support. All the nurses wanted to serve his room. Sushil was worried that the mass copying of his poem there might result in plagiarism. He later got all Divyansh's poems protected with copyright in India.

Dr Ching, the head of the ICU of the hospital, was a competent doctor and a compassionate person. He often told his interns to do research to find a solution for this young man when he visited Divyansh's room for his examination. 'If there is any solution in medical science for this condition, go and find out, we will try it on him,' he said. The US medical system is inflexible. If treatment of any disease was not FDA approved, doctors refrained from trying new treatments on patients. Dr Ching, in the same prevailing restriction, was willing to try all treatment options which could potentially hold promise for Divyansh.

Dr James Mac visited Divyansh in the ICU. He generally expressed his disappointment at his deteriorating condition. Sushil had a lot of questions to ask him. Without mincing words, he told the doctor, 'You have been examining him for the last six months. We always consulted you when instances of neuro-seizure were exhibited by Divyansh. You always said that this was the side effects of drugs. Did you ever make out that this could be necrotizing encephalitis caused by Methotrexate toxicity? If the answer to this question is, yes, then why did you continue giving him intrathecal Methotrexate even thereafter every month?' The questions were so direct and fact-based that the doctor initially replied to him vaguely, saying that his medical condition was rare and different patients responded differently to this treatment. Sushil was not the least bit satisfied with his answer. He concluded that either the doctor had ignorantly allowed the symptoms to worsen or didn't have knowledge that Methotrexate-induced toxicity could take such menacing proportions. Before the doctor left, Sushil told him that had he allowed his brain biopsy at the first instance of seizure, as the neuro-oncologist had suggested, we would have explored the possibility of treating him with hyperbaric oxygen chamber. Now, even that option was gone. All through Divyansh's treatment in the past eight years, we had always been vigilant about new symptoms showing up in Divyansh. We reported immediately to the doctors without wasting even a day—such was our alertness. What could we do if the doctor for reasons best known to him acted like this? We could allow some discount to the doctor because Divyansh's case was a difficult one, reporting repeated relapse, even after transplantation. But acting on time to tackle new symptoms that could be potentially threatening was in the hands of the doctor.

We were still clueless as to how intrathecal Methotrexate could result in so much toxicity leading to necrotizing effect. Divyansh was earlier given this treatment after his first relapse in 2012 which continued till transplantation, and there were no such instances during that period. Sushil was working on the answer to this crucial question in order to explore any possible treatment.

But we began asking ourselves the question: what was Divyansh's future if there were no treatment options left for him except support treatment? Thus began the quests for doctors from whom a second opinion could be obtained.

Sushil began searching for a neuro-oncologist who could be contacted for a second opinion. At that time, Khush came to be with us for some days. He helped a lot in the search process.

Finally, we zeroed in on a doctor named Fredrick (pseudonym) at a New York-based hospital. Somehow, Sushil contact him over the phone. He was ready to see Divyansh but he would have to be brought to his clinic, which was not possible. He couldn't have come to see him in the hospital Divyansh was in. With great reluctance, he agreed to see his MRI CD. Sushil delivered it to his clinic. He was promised that Dr Fredrick would call him after seeing it.

Meanwhile, Sushil contacted the doctor at the hospital in Texas who had treated Divyansh with Methotrexate via email and asked his advice on any possible treatment for this medical condition. To our astonishment, he curtly replied that he didn't have any experience in dealing with leukoencephalopathy. Sushil wrote back requesting him to ascertain from other departments or doctors in his hospital if they could suggest any treatment plan. Shockingly, the doctor didn't reply to this mail. We lost all hope of hearing from him.

Meanwhile, Divyansh's pneumonic patch gradually improved. The doctor planned to wean him off the life support.

❧

20

WE WILL WITHSTAND ALL TOGETHER

Since we had come to USA, Divyansh waited for the day when he would see the first snowfall of his life. The East Coast of USA is known for its excessively cold weather and snowfall from December to February. In the past, we had been to Kashmir to see the wonder of nature's snow-clad mountains. But we were not fortunate enough to see the snow falling. It was the second week of December in New Jersey. As we set out in the morning from Ajay's home to be with Divyansh in the ICU, we witnessed heavy snowfall all the way. I was transported to the serene tranquillity of Pahalgam where Divyansh had wished to see snowfall live. Today was the day. I didn't know that snowfall could be so teasing and painful to see when it finally happened in my life. When we reached Divyansh's room, the city was still experiencing heavy snowfall, which was clearly visible through the glass window of his ICU room. The snowfall was real, but to me, it appeared illusory. I couldn't fathom any beauty in it that even I had waited to see. It surely didn't bring the happiness that Divyansh had wished to soak himself in. I only wished it brought the warmth of spring into Divyansh's life when it finally went away.

In two weeks' time, Divyansh was weaned off life support after his condition improved, and was shifted to the step-down ICU, which is nothing but a semi-ICU set-up, though the latest MRI scan of the brain didn't reveal any improvement in the lesions.

For me, the step-down ICU was much better, away from the constant buzzing sounds of the ICU monitors, and here I could be with Divyansh in his room full time. All through this, my own condition was worsening. My appetite had gone down. Anxiety and stress caused me to fall down in the hospital. My existential value in my own eyes had become worth a peanut. It must have been tough for Sushil to manage me and Divyansh, along with doing research for a possible treatment option for him. Today, as I look back, I can only empathize with him for all the pains and tribulations he went through like me but didn't have a shoulder to lean on. Commendably, whenever he met doctors, nurses or visitors, he made sure to meet them with a smile on his face. Sushil's personality was such that he would share his pain only with a select few he was comfortable with. Unlike me, in the toughest of times, he displayed remarkable equanimity. For him, like Divyansh, pain and suffering were personal, and so they attached a great degree of maintaining their dignity.

When Divyansh was shifted to the ICU, we went back to Ajay's home for the night. When he was in the general ward, Sushil and I stayed with him round the clock, but there was restriction on staying at night in the ICU. While we were in the general ward, I had vowed to go back to Ajay's home only with Divyansh, not without him. Time painfully made me reconcile with my pledge. When we reached his home late at night, I abhorred my condition. Each and every moment reminded me of the negativity my son had to experience in the past couple of months, despite Ajay's best efforts. Sensing this, Sushil searched for a rented apartment near the hospital. It didn't take too much time and he found a decent one just half a kilometre from the hospital. When Sushil discussed with Ajay our plan to shift to a rented accommodation, surprisingly, he didn't say no, but instantly agreed. Yes, the writing on the wall was clear. But how could we shift at a time Divyansh was in the ICU? We, however, went ahead with the agreement to take the apartment on rent, and waited for Divyansh to get a little better before we shifted.

We were fast approaching Christmas Day. The whole city was decorated and in a festive mood. Ajay used to say that Divyansh would surely be fine and discharged from the hospital by Christmas, so he would decorate his house only after he returned from the hospital. Now, that became a remote possibility. I remembered Divyansh's note which he had written in the hospital in December 2009 when he was first diagnosed with leukaemia, which he wondered what gift Santa Claus would bring him on Christmas Day. On this Christmas Day too, I wondered what gift Santa would give my son. Divine gifts are always with us in plenty. What we need to do is realize their presence amidst us with the wisdom we possess, and I had learnt this after reading Divyansh's reflections in December 2009. The only gift from Santa I could visualize this time for Divyansh was complete freedom from his incessant misery or salvation.

The college authority of FDU was responsive to Divyansh's need. By that time, he had missed his first semester examination. They said he would be allowed to join in the second semester and, alongside, clear the pending papers of the first semester. At Christmas time, students were expected to vacate their dorms. This condition couldn't be waived even for Divyansh. In any case, we were not sure when Divyansh would return to the college considering the condition he was in. Ajay drove Sushil and me to Divyansh's dorm to clear out his belongings. His room was tidy; everything was in its appropriate place. Even small stationery was in its designated place. As I began packing his clothes, shoes, bed sheets, toiletries, stationary, etc., I remembered how I myself had assiduously arranged them with my own hands just few months back, and now, the same hands were undoing that. I had arranged his room in his presence with great affection. Now, I was dismantling them in his absence. How would he feel if he saw me uprooting him from his dorm in his absence? Divyansh had earned his place in the campus with great difficulty. Thinking of all this, I was engulfed in a shrieking emotional tide that wrecked me completely. I couldn't hold myself and I fell. When I came to my senses after a few minutes, I held myself with a conviction that I would soon arrange his dorm again in a few days. All the while, I was reminded of his resolve penned in his poem 'The Tree of Purity', which he had written for me on Mother's Day:

> We will withstand all together,
> We will enjoy the spring,
> We will bear our wondrous fruits,
> And be the wonder we are.

In the first week of January 2018, my younger sister, Shikha, joined us to lend a hand. Since Divyansh was shifted to the ICU, she was herself taken ill and desperately wanted to see and be with Divyansh, even though that forced her to leave her eight-year-old son to the care of her husband, Arvind. Actually, Sushil too, considering my own condition of stress and anxiety, wanted her to join us to give me emotional support, even though I never wanted her to come leaving behind her son. My pain and misery would only go with the recovery of Divyansh. Back in Mumbai, my parents and Ananya were in constant touch with us. When they called to know about Divyansh, more often than not, I avoided talking to them because I didn't have anything to share. I didn't want to inflict on them my morose and withdrawn mental condition.

Sushil's and Ajay's indefatigable efforts finally bore results. They accessed a research paper of a US hospital that had successfully treated a patient suffering from acute leukoencephalopathy. We showed these papers to Dr Ching and the neuro-onco-physician Dr Sam Lerman. Dr Ching, despite this being an experimental treatment, agreed to try it on Divyansh, whereas the neuro-onco-physician felt that this might not work. We prevailed upon him on the premise that in any case, they were not treating Divyansh with any proven treatment plan; there was no harm in trying this, especially when it had worked in one acute case. Incidentally, this research paper was from the same hospital in Texas where Divyansh had undergone treatment, and the doctor there, despite repeated request from us earlier on, didn't bother to check with his own facility. The experimental treatment protocol was a combination of three drugs to be administered for 15 days. We didn't want to omit anything which might work on Divyansh. Dr Ching felt it was worth trying as well. He too, like us, always felt that Divyansh was a young person, and they must not leave any stone unturned in getting him back to his life. Subconsciously, we were racing against time since the doctor had drawn a timeline for Divyansh. Perseverance and exploring new avenues of treatment— that's what remained in our hands.

27 January 2018, Divyansh's twenty-first birthday. Since a day before, I was scared at the very idea of celebrating it in the step-down ICU, though the nurses were buoyed about it and wanted to make it a big day for him. He was not in his complete senses. It would be painful for me to make him hold a knife in his hand and force him to cut a cake mechanically. Sushil, on the other hand, thought to give it new meaning with some unexpected people who came into his life by divine design. He felt Divyansh's birthday was not only for us, but also for them. He ordered for a big cake a day before. The next morning, we reached his room with the cake but without a gift for him for the first time in his entire life. This poor mother had only her blessings and prayers to gift him, nothing less and nothing more. To our surprise, we found the room decorated with colourful balloons and cut-outs. But the bigger surprise came from Susan as she arrived when we were just about to cut the cake. Talking about gifts, yes, she came with a gift. Divyansh himself was the chief reason for that

gift, very thoughtfully conceived and executed by Susan. As she unwrapped the gift, I couldn't hold back my tears. She had taken prints of all his blog articles by painstakingly downloading them from his blog wall, meticulously labelled them, made an index page, and put them in a box-file with the title, 'Reflections of Divyansh Atman'. The whole event as it panned out was surreal to us. That day, I realized what a gift actually meant. I don't know how much of it was for Divyansh but it helped me recalibrate my thoughts and celebrate his birthday with some gusto.

The box-file found a permanent place in his room. Nurses and doctors visiting his room would often flip through its pages, read a few and gesture their amazement before leaving. Many a time, nurses would take it to the nursing station to read quietly when they were at leisure. Divyansh's way of impacting their lives was perceivable even though he was not communicating.

At the time, Dr Ching agreed to start the experimental treatment on Divyansh, he had to again be shifted to the ICU for the same reason: aspiration in the lungs and a sharp drop in oxygen saturation. He was again intubated and put on life support. The nurses who had earlier served him were shocked to see him there again. The kind of love they had for Divyansh was juxtaposed with what love is normally perceived from me. They didn't want to see Divyansh in the ICU in close proximity to them, forcing them to serve him again. They wished to see him away from them. In a short period of time, their presence in the ICU room became sublime to us, where they often appeared to be stepping into my shoes and I, quietly and invisibly, lay by Divyansh's side, to receive their emotional balm.

Anyway, the experimental treatment began. We had our fingers crossed. Meanwhile, Dr Fredrick from New York, after a lot of persuasion, called Sushil to meet him. We were waiting for his appointment as we wanted to know the accuracy of the prognosis the doctors of the hospital had made, and if there was still any treatment option left to be tried.

Sushil and Ajay went to meet him with all Divyansh's medical records and the most recent MRI scan CD. Dr Fredrick was a young and tall person, in his late 30s, who didn't believe in being verbose when making a medical point. After going through Divyansh's medical case history, all the treatments given at various stages and the latest MRI scan, said, 'Look Mr Sushil, I am a neuro-oncologist. Which means I am neurologist first and oncologist later. It's very unfortunate for me to say that the medical reports of your son are not good. What I understand is that after the transplantation, more specifically, after radiation at the time of transplantation, the condition of his brain changed. After the CNS relapse this time, had you approached me, I would have told you to take a considered decision with the neurological aspects in mind. That would have been: if we go ahead with intrathecal Methotrexate, the brain might be a victim of toxicity and we don't know what happens after that. And if we leave this untreated then you know what's going to happen. When the doctor at the Texas hospital prescribed the treatment by Methotrexate in a radiated brain, he should have discussed its pros and cons, and after that, it should have been left to you to take an appropriate decision. In any case, if they decided to go ahead with this treatment, they should have set a protocol to periodically check the condition of the brain by MRI scan, so long as the treatment by intrathecal Methotrexate was underway. They didn't do so, which rendered the deteriorating conditions of the brain unnoticed for a long time. When you brought your son to the New Jersey-based hospital, they too, despite repeated instances of neuro-seizures, didn't consider it necessary to do periodical MRIs. Possibly they didn't anticipate the toxicity had begun taking an irreversible toll. Whatever has happened with your son is a rare phenomenon reported in very few medical journals. But maybe a case like this could trigger us to do more research on the treatment of these medical conditions for such patients in the future. However, the experimental treatment based on a medical journal that you have got started holds some promise. Good luck.'

We now had the true picture. Knowing fully well that there was no more treatment option left for my son, the doctors in Texas and later in New Jersey should have gone ahead with Methotrexate with caution, as felt by Dr Fredrick. The best recourse, however, was to wait for the disease to come back so that Divyansh could have become eligible for the trial treatment. While these thoughts frustrated our minds making us feel helpless, a lady doctor of Indian origin visited Divyansh in the ICU in the absence of Dr Ching and dispassionately said to us that his chances of survival were very grim. Sushil couldn't hold it any more, especially after listening to Dr Fredrick earlier on. He retorted:

> You are a doctor. I know medical science has its limitations. But it evolves every day. The opinion you hold for my son is based on the knowledge you possess as of date. Someone may have better knowledge than you. Maybe your own knowledge can be improved upon when you go back to your home today or in days to come. Since you also come from India, I would expect you to do your karma. Explore all avenues. You have neither given birth to my son nor can you become a cause of his death. I am going to support in all your endeavours to figure out any possible treatment for my son. I am not a person with a medical background. But by dint of my resolute efforts, I could find an experimental treatment which was tried successfully in such medical conditions. Please do that rather than forecasting the death of your patients.

The doctor, listening to Sushil's outburst, was bowled over. She hadn't expected this. Without saying anything more, she talked to the nurses, gave them some instructions and hurriedly left the department. I was quite relieved to hear Sushil speak his mind. He dared to question the approach of the doctor. The next day, the first thing the doctor said to Sushil, after she arrived was, 'I am sorry.'

Divyansh's condition improved as the pneumonic patch in his lungs dissipated. He was weaned off life support. By then, the experimental treatment was also over. The nurses were happy to shift him to the step-down ICU again. Divyansh was better this time as compared to his earlier discharge from ICU. His facial responses looked more alive. He seemed to be trying to connect with us.

The hospital had a healthy practice of engaging a priest from the Chapel attached to the hospital with each patient. The priest, a man in his late 50s, visited Divyansh, in the general ward, the ICU and the step-down ICU almost daily, barring weekends. When he came, he talked to us for some time and then expected us to leave the room for a couple of minutes to allow him to pray for Divyansh without any distraction. I observed that there invariably was a smile on his face after he was done with his prayers. Our hospital stay by then had been over two months. In these two months, whatever communication the priest had with Divyansh was only non-verbal. As days passed by, his attachment to Divyansh grew deeper. That non-verbal communication from a placid person could be so powerful and overwhelming—I witnessed with my own eyes. The priest was certainly spending more time with him as compared to the other patients. One day, after Divyansh was admitted to the step-down ICU for the second time after the experimental treatment, as usual, the priest came and stood by Divyansh's bedside for five minutes. With his characteristic smile on his face, he emerged from the room after praying for him. That day, I asked him for the first time his reflections on Divyansh and if he would improve in the coming days. He listened to me attentively, looked at Divyansh from outside his room where we stood, was silent for a while and finally said:

> I have been visiting your son for a long time. His soul attracts
> me. When I stand by his side, I don't feel like leaving him.
> I must tell you, though your son is hardly 21 years old, his
> soul is maybe that of a 50-year-old. It reflects miraculous
> energy to me as I stand near him. Its effect is overpowering
> on me. I get the feeling that he always tries to communicate
> with me through the energy radiated by his soul. It seems
> his soul is in his complete command and he actually makes
> me feel its profoundness. The kind of impression I get from
> his soul makes me feel that his survival or non-survival is
> in his hands, no matter how much we try. I would advise
> you to trust the wisdom of your son and his soul. Whatever
> he does, must be good for all of us. I guess it is between
> him and God now.

With these words, he blessed me and left to see a patient in the
adjacent room. I sat quietly in a corner chair and remembered
the time of Divyansh's birth in Patna, with the blessed soul the
priest was talking about.

⁂

21

HIS NAME PERSONIFIES HIM

I was in USA on a tourist visa. It was about six months since I had come here. The rules required a person on a tourist visa to stay for not more than six months at a time. I was forced to return to India for a week to comply with the visa conditions. It was tough for me to leave Divyansh in the hospital and travel to India. Most of the establishments in USA work on a binary system: yes or no. There was nothing between the yes and no that would help me continue to stay there considering Divyansh's medical condition. It was pointless to make a petition to the Department of Homeland Security for an extended stay, as they would have, in all likelihood, rejected the prayer. It was more sensible to go to India for a week and then come back.

My body returned to India while my soul remained with Divyansh. As I embarked on the flight completely disoriented and made my way to my seat, I felt like crying without caring for my fellow passengers. But in the end, only motionless tears accompanied me on the journey. The excitement of meeting Ananya after six months was completely eclipsed by the enormity of pain of leaving Divyansh in the hospital.

On reaching home in Mumbai, there was no excitement at meeting Ananya and my parents after such a long time. I was just waiting for my day of departure again. Sushil and Shikha called me twice a day. Sometimes he made me talk to Divyansh on video chat. Sushil told me that Divyansh looked a little improved, though I didn't notice anything of this sort during the video call. He was probably just trying to keep me in good spirits as I was preparing to return to New Jersey.

Disembarking from the flight, when I presented myself to the immigration authority at the airport in New Jersey, they refused to give me clearance, stating that I had been visiting USA quite regularly since March last year on a tourist visa. Despite my best efforts to convince them of my son's hospitalization, they were not ready to clear my immigration. They threatened to deport me. I got agitated at the thought of not being with Divyansh if they did that. Sushil, who had come to the airport to receive me, kept calling me to know the status of my clearance from the immigration kiosk. I was not able to take his call as using mobile phones in the immigration hall was strictly prohibited. Finally, after a lot of persuasion, I was taken to a higher-up in immigration. He saw the hospital papers and was sympathetic to my plight. He quickly cleared the immigration and wished me good luck. That one hour of confusion and constant threats of deporting me to India was so torturous and frustrating that I felt like fighting with him. I felt like screaming at them and saying, 'Go check my son's condition in the hospital.' But in the end, good sense prevailed and I was allowed to go out. Sushil waited anxiously for me at the arrival gate. He said that had they decided to deport me, there was nothing we could have done.

I was reunited with my soul when I met Divyansh after seven days of separation.

Divyansh was definitely looking better. His expressions were alive. We supposed the experimental treatment had some effect on him. The doctors and nurses in the ICU constantly visited him to see his recovery. They were happy to see a miracle dawning. What moved me was that Divyansh, seeing me after a gap of seven days, began to cry. This expression was a happy surprise for us. It meant he was trying to connect with us. It is ironic: for the first time, a mother was glad when her son cried. Sushil handled Divyansh's emotional outburst and my gleam with a felicitous remark, 'Divyansh, this time too, you will make it.' While we soaked ourselves in the new hope Divyansh had showered on us, Susan entered the room. Divyansh again cried in the same manner when Susan talked to him. Sushil expected an encouraging response from her as she witnessed this new development. But she had something else to say. She looked at us and said candidly, 'Maybe, he wants to tell you to let him…'. She purposely left the incomplete sentence hanging and looked affectionately at Divyansh. She wanted us to realize what she had tried to convey. While in the ICU, we saw some cases where the doctors and patients' caregivers allowed the patients to pass away when their conditions worsened beyond the scope of any recovery. It was shocking to us to see family members like husbands, parents or siblings allowing the doctor to cut the lifeline of their patients, namely, their own dear ones. Was Susan hinting at this? We simply got rid of this shocking proposition when she left the room and continued reliving the new hope Divyansh had given us.

It was time for us to pack our bags and leave Ajay's home. The mere act of entering his house late every night when we returned from the hospital had become demoralizing for me. His family undoubtedly tried to help us initially. Our extended stay there for reasons beyond our control and Ajay's growing affinity with Divyansh perhaps created the difference. The day we left his home for good, I was relieved. The suffering which had taken a toll on my dignity, was alleviated. I felt Divyansh's and my self-respect was redeemed. The rented apartment that we had taken near the hospital was spacious and well-located. In no time, we set up our apartment and could attend to Divyansh from a closer location.

Ajay had to travel on a business trip to India, China and Japan in early March 2018. He was due to go for on a similar trip last December, but postponed it considering Divyansh's critical conditions then. Dr Ulrich Rohde, his boss, was kind enough to exempt him from the trip to enable him to devote his attention to Divyansh. Ajay could not request him to postpone his visit again this time. I sensed that he himself wanted to go. Sushil told him to go ahead with his visit. In any case, we had shifted to the rented apartment by that time and it was not a problem to manage things on our own in his absence. And though Sushil initially apprehended some problems, they didn't materialize. Sushil had been involved in Divyansh's day-to-day medical management in the hospital and out of the hospital as well since Divyansh was hospitalized in the third week of November last year.

Sushil's eldest brother, Shankar Bhaiya, joined us in the second week of March. He came to see Divyansh and to be with us for a month. Bhaiya is a retired government servant who maintains a strict discipline for himself. With his brother joining him, Sushil was relieved as there were times he needed to share his emotions with someone he was comfortable with.

In American hospitals, there is an inhuman system of dumping the patients or forcing them to get discharged once the hospitals concluded there was no treatment for their medical conditions. The hospitals there work under immense pressure from insurance industries that keep tabs on the ongoing treatments and billings of the patients' treatment. The hospitals invariably get pinched by these companies when they think the continuance of the patients' treatment in the hospital is unnecessary. The hospitals are always mindful of this cardinal principle while treating difficult cases. Some of the hospitals there were also directly or indirectly owned by insurance companies, and so the unholy practice continues unabated.

We became victims of this practice. We began to feel the pressure from the hospital to discharge our son and look for a rehabilitation centre for Divyansh. It was a rude shock to us. Divyansh was in no condition to be discharged. Ajay was away on his business tour. Sushil individually met the management and tried to convince them to review the decision but in vain. Finally, with no help in sight, he met the patient advocacy of the hospital and narrated the problem. He officially wrote a mail to the advocacy citing negligence and error of judgement of the treating oncologist in continuing with Methotrexate and delaying the diagnosis. The mail worked because the management feared it might take a medico-legal turn, though we had no intention to make it that. It was a question of Divyansh's dignity, which we couldn't allow to be subject to pity and discarded by the hospital. So, we continued thereafter.

However, with time, we realized that continuing in the hospital was not in Divyansh's interest. He actually needed a rehab facility where his day-to-day medical needs and therapies could be attended to more vigorously. The experimental treatment had its shelf-life. The latest MRI scan of the brain did not show any improvement. While we looked for a good rehab around the hospital, I felt the need to do one more thing before leaving the hospital. I wanted to talk to the oncologist Dr James Mac, who had been treating Divyansh since we came to New Jersey. I got a chance to speak to him the very next day when he came to see a patient in the room next to Divyansh. Nurses flocked around him. I requested for time alone to talk to him. He readily agreed. He finished with his patients, called me to the other end of the department and generally spoke about Divyansh's worsening condition.

I said, 'Can a mother say something to you? I expect you to give me a patient hearing till I conclude.' He said yes.

'Doctor, I have been thinking to tell you something for the last three months. Now, since we have decided to move to a rehab, let me tell you this. Apart from his fate, you are responsible for Divyansh's present medical condition,' I unhesitatingly spoke out my darkest sorrow.

He was stunned. He didn't expect this would come to him

in such a direct way. With a wide grin on his face, he asked me what made me think that about him.

'Please consider the pain of a mother. We came to you from day one with a lot of hope. You ignored his symptoms and kept injecting him with Methotrexate which itself was the cause of his deteriorating condition. Your sheer ignorance of his symptoms for a long time, maybe unknowingly, allowed his condition to worsen, dragging him to a point of no return. You have ruined my son's life and mine too,' I reiterated.

He interrupted, 'If you don't trust me, I can put you on to a different doctor.'

'No doctor, don't make another doctor suffer the mess created by you. I have been choked by these thoughts for a long time. I just wanted to release them to you before leaving the hospital,' I finished with a sigh.

The doctor was dumbfounded. He immediately left the place in a huff, fearing embarrassment as the nurses had started gathering around.

I felt relieved and moved on towards Divyansh's room nonchalantly.

Sushil had been in USA since last November, more than four months away from his office. His leave had expired long ago. He was extending it every fortnight. His boss was an outstanding human being to say the least. He never allowed the pressure of the office to build up on him while he was in USA with us. But there were some pressing matters which required him to join his office as early as possible. Time had always subjected him to strenuous tests in his life. And every time, he did what he thought was the right thing to do at that juncture. He decided to take a break for a month or two to attend to his office demands and then come back here again. We had finalized a rehab facility close to the hospital. Around the end of March when Sushil planned to leave for Mumbai, we decided to move Divyansh to the rehab facility.

By that time, Ajay was expected to be back from his business visit. Bhaiya, too, rose to the occasion and agreed to extend his stay with us till Sushil came back from Mumbai. Honestly, I too wanted Sushil to take a small break. For the last four months, I had painfully watched him exhausting himself every day without complaint and with a smile on his face. He was adept at multi-tasking. He was managing Divyansh, me, Ananya's studies and his office work whilst in USA. I was worried that his resilient endurance would weaken if he continued like this. I had become proficient in Divyansh's medical management and was confident I could manage everything on my own in his absence. Shikha too had left to get back to her family in India.

But it wasn't so simple for Sushil to leave Divyansh when he needed him all the time. It was a tough call he had to take, which he did considering all the factors. In hindsight, his decision to go back to India for some time helped us take an even greater decision when he returned with a new idea. Before leaving for the airport, Sushil caressed Divyansh's head with teary eyes, perhaps saying sorry to him. He was choked because he suspected Divyansh would not have liked him to go, leaving him in the hospital. I was sure Divyansh would have understood Sushil's predicament, as I remembered these lines from Divyansh's poem on him, 'His Name Personifies Him':

> This might sound very 'ordinary',
> To a person who is not aware,
> Of the trials and tribulations,
> In his daily life.
> What if I were to tell you, my friends,
> Of his responsibilities,
> Steep as the mountains they are?
> Of the predicaments and misfortunes,
> That have struck him all at once, like thunder and
> lightning?

22

AS A CANDLE'S IN A STORM

We planned to leave the hospital for the rehab facility on 2 April 2018. The hospital attached two nurses to accompany Divyansh all the way to the rehab and inform the medical team there of the details of his discharge summary. The ambulance was waiting for us at the portico. So far, I had only seen an ambulance from a distance. The very sight of them scared me, thinking of the critical conditions of the patients they carry. This was the day I was forced to break my ambulance fright. Ajay and Bhaiya were with me but avoided getting into the ambulance. Missing Sushil badly, I stepped into it with nervousness. The nervousness was more for Divyansh as he was leaving the hospital. I was not sure if he would be properly taken care of in the rehab in the manner he required. I cried mutely. The nurses, engrossed, read Divyansh's medical history and talked aplenty about his mental fortitude all the way. My eyes stopped seeing outside and became blank as the ambulance sped to our destination.

Unlike India, there was a mushrooming growth of rehabilitation centres all over USA. They primarily catered to the needs of older people, who didn't stay with their children for cultural reasons. In our country, old parents live with their sons in most cases, and daughters in some, and there are hardly any such centres here. Besides this, in USA, during their recovery phase, several patients, not requiring intensive treatment in hospitals are sent to the rehab centres for recovery, much to the delight of insurance companies, to reduce the medical expenses of such patients. There are two types of rehab centres operating there: acute rehab centres and sub-acute rehab centres. Divyansh was to be admitted in a sub-acute rehab, where medical treatment was given at a sub-acute level, the main focus being intensive therapy to rehabilitate patients.

We reached the rehab by noon. Divyansh was given a big single-occupancy room with a double bed. The arrangements were fine. The nurses and support staff were helpful and affable. It was painful to see that Divyansh was the only young person amongst the occupants of the rehab, most of who were old people. It ripped my heart and I was nauseated, thinking this could not be a place for my son to stay. However, all these gentle old people came to see him one by one and tried to make me comfortable in whatever way they could. They were quite sympathetic to him.

We were not allowed to stay with Divyansh at night. Leaving him alone there on the first night, when I didn't know or hadn't tested anyone there, was unsettling for me. Around 9 p.m., I saw an assistant practising nurse (APN) in a light blue dress sitting at the door to Divyansh's room. I asked her name. She gently said, 'I am Helen, APN. I know you worry about leaving your son alone as this is your first day here. As it is, we are required to take care of patients all night long. However, please rest assured that I will be sitting all night in your son's room. Please take my mobile number and call me whenever you feel like. I have your mobile number. In case I need to talk, I will call.' It was like a thirsty person hitting a spring to quench his thirst. Before I could thank her, she interrupted me and continued, 'Your son is like my grandson. I will take care of him like that. Now, please go back to your apartment and rest. You seem very tired today. God willing, your son will recover.'

Returning to the apartment, I could only picture Helen, her

angelic persona and Divyansh, getting motherly care from her.

As time progressed in the rehab, we began getting comfort from the place. All the nurses came to know about Divyansh's inspirational journey and his creative and academic excellence. I narrated to them his life story with some pride and they were awed. Gradually, Divyansh became their blue-eyed darling they all wanted to serve. They flocked around him just to say hello. To my surprise, in time, I was known there as Divyansh's mother. My own identity was subsumed in him, even though he was not communicating. The nurses would request the head nurse to allot Divyansh's room for their duty. When some of them failed in their attempt, they came to me complaining about it and to say hello to Divyansh. Of them, the most affectionate service to Divyansh was by Helen. She normally came in to see Divyansh at 3 p.m. as she always had the evening shift. Apart from the medical care and maintaining his body hygiene, she prayed for him for about half an hour. During the hour she spent with Divyansh at the beginning of her shift, she assumed all his responsibility, relieving me from my mental preoccupation with him. The level of her relationship with Divyansh was beyond my comprehension. It seemed like she had some past life connection with Divyansh where she tried to continue from where she might have left. This was another dot Divyansh's life thread seemed to try to join.

One nurse visited Divyansh almost daily, irrespective of the room she was allotted for the day. She came and sat with him, generally talking about things he may have liked. After few days, she stopped coming. I thought she was not coming to the rehab anymore. But I saw her serving a patient in a room downstairs. I met her and said hello. She was happy to see me. I casually asked her if everything was alright as I was meeting her after a week. She candidly confessed to me with tears in her eyes that she was very attached to Divyansh and would often pray for him in Church. But she realized that too much of an emotional attachment to Divyansh didn't augur well for her professional ethics. So she decided to snap her ties with him. But the tears in her eyes still betrayed her battle with professional ethics.

Apart from the medication prescribed by the hospital in its discharge summary, the various therapies given here were intense. The therapists were competent and compassionate. With them, I too learnt the skills of therapy, which I did for Divyansh in their absence. Divyansh's face was alive now. He interacted only through facial expressions. But that was enough to lift the sagging spirits of a mother. I would invoke in myself the spirit he tried to convey in his poem 'Blaze'.

> And rekindle the fire in you,
> To make the spirit strong.

Seeing my dedication, the therapists visiting Divyansh taught me the finer nuances of their practices. I boosted my spirit only through him. Every day, I aimed to better my best of the previous day, hoping it would work on Divyansh. In due course of time, the therapists grew attached to him and to me as well. The emotional connect with which they worked on him was discernible. After their sessions were done, they sat with me and discussed Divyansh's life journey so far and tried to cheer us up.

I was never as passionate about listening to music as Sushil and Divyansh. In order to give him neurological stimulation, I began taking interest in Divyansh's playlist and played him tracks from the list regularly. I don't know how much those tracks stimulated him, but they enlivened my spirit, which made me feel as if Divyansh was listening to them through me. Music was bridging the physical gap between a son and his mother.

Before leaving for Mumbai, Sushil painstakingly briefed his brother Shankar on Divyansh's medical history in great detail and the line of treatment presently going on. All his life, Bhaiya was Sushil's idol. He was just like his father. In fact, I found a lot of similarities in their personalities. Sushil always considered him a bankable person. He expected him to step into his shoes till he returned and to take care of Divyansh and give me emotional support. Astonishingly, Bhaiya remained passive towards his role in Divyansh's treatment process and was much too occupied with his own daily chores. Maybe he couldn't muster enough confidence to deal with his medical issues and day-to-day management in USA. I give him the benefit of the doubt on this. But even remaining passive, he could have let me know that he felt my pain and his mere presence would have been enough to propel me forward with the right spirit. Unfortunately, that didn't happen. Though he was always present physically, he was greatly unmindful of all that was going on with Divyansh. If at all he was mindful, his passive responses hurt me more than helped my cause. There were times I found him painfully insensitive towards a grieving mother and her sick son. I felt helpless. I thought that had I been alone I would have been better placed to manage without any such affliction. I miserably tried to dissemble my loss of faith in him. Even Sushil in Mumbai was helpless as Bhaiya had extended his stay acting on Sushil's wishes only. At the end of the day, I shouldn't blame him for his limitations. The world is full of suffering, yet it is full of people overcoming of them too. His inactions or passive actions made me more stout-hearted to explore ways to deal with my problems.

As Neil Strauss said, 'Great things never came from comfort zones.'

The quintessential Divyansh epitomized this thought. He unfailingly challenged the outer limits of his comfort zones, stretching them outward to accommodate his growing appetite to accomplish what he aspired to. He had been in the hospital since November last. His closest pals, Mridul and Anshoo, couldn't make themselves available at his side when he needed them the most. I can't say if Divyansh still expected them to come and boost his sinking life, but yes, I did. Not because I didn't understand their own personal pressing engagements, though. Anshoo was newly married and just settled into his new corporate life. Mridul, too, apart from his engagement with his corporate life, was recently blessed with an adorable son, and he must have felt some difficulty in leaving them alone in Dubai and travelling to USA to visit Divyansh. Whatever they did, therefore, was well within the comfort zones of their lives. They couldn't challenge it. True self-discovery begins where your comfort zone ends. In the past, they had challenged their comfort zones and often be a part of Divyansh and our painful journey. I guessed they had reached the saturation point of enduring in their relationship with us. They had their own lives. But one thing is sure. While life gives you umpteen chances to redeem your faith, glory and missed opportunities, a time comes when you no longer get one. That's a big full stop. I believed they had hit this full stop. If you are sensitive enough, you may have a sense of remorse at a later stage in life, otherwise you are just like any normal human being, enjoying the security of comfort zones. During the time we were in rehab, Anshoo came to Seattle for a business trip. On completion of his official assignment, he did drop in on us for a day before travelling back to India. More than me, Anshoo knew he was absently present for Divyansh that day. Perhaps, Divyansh knew too. Painfully, the two closest pals, despite their physical presence together, were absent for each other that day. My painful reflection about them is only to underscore a point that of all the kids at my in-laws' place, I cared for and loved them the most. We were in a terribly difficult situation here. They couldn't have done anything to improve it. What they could have done was to boost my spirit with their physical presence or even live presence from their absence. I say this because for the last nine years, the greatest mental support I had been getting was from Divyansh only, to help him challenge his comfort zone and ours as well. Now when Divyansh was down, I, unknowingly, was looking at them.

Whilst these old relationships were being subjected to the test of time, silently, new people were finding ways to touch Divyansh's life. One such person was Malina, an occupant at the rehab, just adjacent to Divyansh's room. She was a short lady, with a wrinkled face and wore thick-framed spectacles. She walked with help of a walker. She could walk without it too, but the doctor had advised her to use it to avoid emergencies. She was in her mid-70s then, a loquacious person who often indulged in bad-mouthing the staff at the rehab. This made her a person to be avoided in the facility, but she cared a damn about it. She was a world within herself, living life on her own terms. With a cigarette in her hand, she looked like an absolutely debonair and happy-go-lucky person. She apparently didn't need anyone at her age. Whenever a nurse passed her by, she said something to offend her. All the staff members had learnt to live with her antics as she remained intransigent to follow the code of the rehab. Seeing all this, I obviously avoided her initially, though she peeped in while passing our room. With time, without any communication and only through the gaze of her eyes, she showed an altogether different side of her personality to us, hitherto unknown to the other occupants and staff of the rehab. One day, she finally made it to my room and said to me, 'Hey Honey, your eyes are very beautiful.' 'But my fate is not good,' I instantly replied. 'Shut up! I will slap you hard,' she said, smiled and walked away. The next day, she came again and expressed her desire to talk to Divyansh and to me. With some inhibition, I reciprocated in the same manner. After spending some time with us, she told me not to bring lunch the next day as she would order a pizza which she wished to share with me. I couldn't say no. The next day, I ate lunch with her as curious onlookers from outside the room watched the rare bonhomie of Malina and an occupant of the rehab. Over the next few weeks, she visited our room almost daily, and the first thing she said was, 'Hello Divyansh! I am Malina, your friend. I have come to see and bless you.' And she prayed for him. These happenings were much to the chagrin of the nurses who wanted to protect Divyansh from an evil person like her. They often advised me to stay away from Malina after she left our room. Every person, no matter how independent or evil they may be, has a softer and vulnerable side. Malina was no exception, and I could sense the soft spots of her personality as I grew closer to her. She would often say that her caring son was coming to give her money that day. He never came. At least, I never saw him as long as I was there. As she had some nagging comorbidity of lungs, she was not supposed to smoke. At my constant pestering, she stopped smoking in my presence. She smoked standing away from the rehab centre, under a banyan tree, to avoid my vigilant eyes. When caught red-handed, she shamelessly said that it was the last one she was smoking. But the last one never came. I, too, began enjoying caring for her. Every day, I cooked some Indian delicacies for her, which she savoured after locking her room from the inside. Whatever food she got from the rehab, she shared with me. Sometimes, she secretly brought me juices and cookies from the dining area and ensured I ate them in her presence. Malina, though an independent and carefree lady by appearance, had a deep, sensitive side that I sensed, which perhaps Divyansh did too, through non-verbal communication, by blowing off the thin veil covering it all round. It simply required a gentle breath to see her inner beauty and she probably found no one to do that.

In the rehab facilities in USA, weekdays are lonesome and cheerless. I was the only person who spent all her time every day of the week there. However, it became colourful on weekends when relatives of the occupants came to visit them, wearing colourful clothes and bringing gifts. I never saw any relatives of Malina ever visit her over weekends. I guess she didn't need any one. Divyansh and I were now there to give her company round the clock.

All the occupants of the rehab had almost common stories. They were old, mostly in their late 60s or 70s, away from their families, with some comorbidity. When Divyansh joined their homogeneous bandwagon, he became a talking point and the centre of discussion among them. They liked to know more about him. One day, an old man in a wheelchair visited our room. I had seen him quite often in the corridor of the rehab visiting his friends in other rooms. His own room was downstairs. He was an extrovert and spoke typical American English. He knocked and asked, 'May I come in?' I said, 'Please come.' After we had introduced ourselves, he wheeled his chair to Divyansh's side and kept looking at him, trying to weave a relationship with him or connect some dots of his own life with him. After some time, he told me he had heard that Divyansh wrote well. He wished to read his articles. Like in the hospital, I used to keep the compilation of his blog articles gifted by Susan on his last birthday here in the rehab room too. I happily shared the box-file with him. I also shared a few of his poems. He said he would like to read them in his room and would return them by evening. He didn't come that evening. I didn't mind that he had not kept his word. However, he came the next morning with the box-file on his lap, wheeling his chair with both hands as he entered our room.

He asked me, 'Which country are you from?' 'India,' I said. He looked surprised and said, 'Oh! I thought your son might not be living in India.' I looked at him with a bewildered expression and replied, 'No, my son has been living in India all along. Yes, since last year, he has been studying in New Jersey, pursuing under-graduation in engineering from FDU. But what made you ask this question?' He replied, 'Please don't take me wrong. I retied as an English teacher from a college. It took me some time to absorb the underlying thoughts in your son's blogs and poems. That's why I couldn't return the compilation yesterday as promised by me. His command over the English language can easily be bracketed with big writers. I myself have been an English teacher. His writing skill amazed me. Please protect them with copyright else they will be victims of plagiarism in USA. The reason I asked about your country was because I was surprised to see an Indian boy writing such quality thoughts with supreme command on the language. Anyway, thanks for sharing this with me. Please don't mind if I come once daily to be with your son for two minutes. It will be my pleasure. And yes, you are blessed to be his parent.' As he left the room, he left an indelible paraph of his wheelchair not only on the floor, but also on my heart.

Since we came to the rehab, I noticed that Ajay was away more and more on business trips. Though he was there with us, visiting daily when he was in the city, I had the feeling that he was now wearing a façade of his seriousness towards us. The unconditional love for Divyansh I had seen in him was seemingly waning. The only reason I could attribute to this was a hopeless situational fatigue as a result of protracted treatment with no hope of getting better. He saw too much promise in Divyansh. He selflessly invested his time and energy to pave a way for him to excel and harness his potential. If after all one had done, Divyansh reached the stage he was in, one would feel dejected, and I understood that. Apart from this, there may have been other factors like his entrapment in the viciousness of our problems, from which he might have thought it would be difficult to extricate himself if we continued to remain in that situation for long. There may also have been some family pressure, I guess, which had affected his bonding with Divyansh. His love and affection for him had come as a divine wish. Now, when it was waning, I could not complain about it. But it pained me to see his mutating relation with Divyansh, forget me as his new-found sister.

Towards mid-May in 2018, Divyansh was again engulfed with some serious infection in his lungs, which the doctor had expected, considering his neurological condition. I was completely clueless about what to do. Ajay advised me against shifting him to the hospital. However, the attending nurse Sara advised me to do what a mother should do. She said, 'I have been observing his deteriorating condition for the last two days. I had gone to the Church yesterday to pray for him. My gut feeling says he must be seen by expert doctors under intensive care. Please take him to the hospital.' Her timely, unambiguous advice helped me make a quick decision. This was also because the rehab was a sub-acute one, and intensive treatment could not have been given. We decided to shift Divyansh in an emergency condition to the same hospital late one night. Since we left the hospital for rehab last month, I never imagined that Divyansh would have to return here yet another time. The sight of him being driven again to the same hospital in an ambulance sickened me. I was traumatized all the way to the hospital, wondering if we would to return to rehab again considering his poor condition. I badly missed Sushil, though we were in constant touch on the phone.

❧

23

STRONG AND MIGHTY, THEY STAND UNAFRAID

Divyansh was first admitted in the ER of the hospital. A battery of doctors encircled him. I listened to them but nothing registered in my mind. For some time, I felt I was entwined with Divyansh. Whatever the ferocious effects of life-threatening infections and the force of nature, I was there with all my motherly might to protect him. I regained my composure in half an hour. Divyansh was taken for various tests. Ajay and Bhaiya joined me. After the tests, Divyansh was shifted first to the ICU, and then to the step-down facility. After seven days of hospitalization, he recovered from the bout of infection and was discharged for rehab care. The very prospect of going back to rehab felt like I was taking him home. Before leaving the hospital, I called Sara and Malina about it. As the ambulance entered the portico of the rehab, I saw Malina puffing a cigarette in a tearing hurry under the banyan tree. No sooner had she seen me that she tried to hide it from my sight unsuccessfully, but came running to hug me with moist eyes. Divyansh and I found solace in our new-found home, and Malina reclaimed her companion for all days of the week. In response to a text message from Sushil as he planned to come to New Jersey, I wrote: 'One thing is sure; I will never give up as long as Divyansh doesn't give up.'

By the end of May, Sushil joined us after taking leave from his office for a couple of months. The idea was to stay with Divyansh as long as he could go on. By the time he came, I had become adept at Divyansh's medical management, especially those related to the rehab, but the very feeling of his presence with me round the clock, was confidence boosting. I noticed a definite change in Divyansh's facial expression when he saw his father after almost two months. Bhaiya, soon after Sushil's arrival, went back to India as planned, since, by then, he had already spent three months with us.

None of the staff members and the occupants of the rehab knew Sushil before, though I had made some of them, including Malina, talk to him on the phone. Almost all the staff members knew in advance that Divyansh's father was coming shortly. It would not be an exaggeration if I said that along with Divyansh and I, they too waited with equal intensity for his arrival. Such was the impact of Divyansh on them that they wanted him to get everything he deserved, including Sushil's unstinting presence with him. Moreover, some of the nurses, therapists and, of course, Malina cared so much for me that they wished to see a smile on my face, which they thought Sushil might bring with his presence. So, his date of arrival was known to all in the rehab and he was welcomed when he finally made it. The first day he stepped into the rehab, he had bought some gifts for some chosen nurses and for Malina. It was an absolute pleasure to give those gifts to my new-found friends there. But more than that, I felt true beatitude when I introduced Sushil as my husband and Divyansh's father to all the staff members. In no time, Sushil became known amongst them for his affable personality. Some of the nurses came especially to see who Divyansh's father and my husband was. Initially, they thought Sushil was a doctor because while accompanying Divyansh for the past nine years, he had picked up medical terms and would often describe his medical journey—past or present—as if he were a doctor. In fact, while discussing updates on Divyansh one day with Sushil, the visiting pulmonologist did ask him if he was a doctor.

Reaching the rehab by 9 a.m. in the morning and staying there till late night became our daily routine. Sushil quickly assessed Divyansh's medical condition, the treatment and other support therapies being given to him and got into the groove to give renewed impetus to put him back on his feet, though the task was daunting. Soon after his arrival, Ajay again proceeded on a long business trip to western USA.

Of all the therapists who attended to Divyansh, two names worth mentioning are Sarah, a young girl, a little older than Divyansh in age. She bonded well with him. Normally, a session lasted 45 minutes. She worked on him for at least an hour and a half. After that, she spent half an hour with me to share my pain and to know more about Divyansh. Divyansh's impact on her was visible. The day her session went well, she was happy. Some days were not good, and so she felt disappointed after the session. She appeared melancholic. She gave her 100 per cent, if not more, to improve Divyansh's condition. Sarah gave me hope. She pushed Divyansh's soul to work even harder when medical science ceased to work.

The other therapist's name was Harold. He was an old man, probably in his late 60s then. He was a bit unorthodox in his profession, where he attempted things that others might not have. He felt Divyansh needed this approach, and he responded well to his sessions. Harold, who had probably seen the world by then, guided me to learn whatever he was applying on Divyansh, so that I could continue doing that whenever I had the time. Undoubtedly, he was giving more arsenal in the quiver of a mother to enhance her might.

I found a definite change in Sushil's thought process this time. He often said that USA no longer held any promise for Divyansh. What he was getting here was only support treatment. Even the doctors looked withdrawn from any real hope of reviving him. But for the empathy and genuine concern for Divyansh from the staff at the rehab, there was nothing they could do to ameliorate his condition. Above all, what disconcerted him was the abject surrender of the doctors, despite Divyansh giving valiant fight to come back, thus showing no respect for his dignity. Their feelings of sympathy or empathy for Divyansh were fine, but the sense of him being (medically) condemned by them was not acceptable to Sushil. Medical science has its own limitations—it can't be overemphasized. But one just couldn't question the spirit of Divyansh's soul with which he was trying to fight back. Allopathic medical science diagnoses ailments and treats them at anatomical level, so it has to remain within the confines of the human anatomy. It can never decipher the prowess of a soul, and that is why we often hear examples of unprecedented fight-back by terminally ill patients, much beyond the comprehension of medical science. With this thought in mind, Sushil gauged my response whether it was a good idea to take Divyansh back to Mumbai to rest in the cosy ambience of home where some alternative treatment could be tried as well. This idea also got cemented as he began to find his only support base, Ajay, more and more away due to business trips.

The days were passing. Some days were good for Divyansh from the point of view of his recovery. Some were bad days too. We were moving along as if time had stopped ticking for us. The day before looked no different from the day after. Sushil was becoming a victim to the monotony of rehab life. However, he tried to break the monotony for us and tried new things for Divyansh every day. Through the day, I consciously kept him away from the various therapy sessions Divyansh underwent in my presence. I tried my best to lessen his stress in the limited way I could. He was subjected to this for years in the past, saving me from strain caused by the complex treatment process. Now was my turn to save him. Our mutual conscious endeavours to save one another from some inevitable pain in different times and space was the reason for our ever-strengthening conjugal bond, which this pain had unwittingly resulted.

In early July, Divyansh's lungs were infected again. The doctors of the rehab advised us to take him to the hospital for acute care. After hospitalization, Divyansh got better within few days of starting treatment. A visit to the hospital in less than a month and a half gave us a wake-up call. Sushil asked the doctor to take his MRI scan to assess if it had got better. The scan didn't show an encouraging picture. Rather, it was worsening. We thought that episodes like this necessitating him to take treatment in the hospital set-up would keep recurring. There seemed no end to it. We had almost hit a dead end. If there was anything which could work for him, it was obviously not through the rigmarole of shuttling between the rehab and the hospital. It was time to think out-of-the-box.

While we were in hospital, Sushil asked me one morning, 'Nidhi, I have been thinking something for the last two days. The time has come to take your advice and comfort into account before moving ahead with this. Look, Divyansh is not getting any concrete treatment for his medical condition of leukoencephalopathy. What he is getting is only support treatment. Our support base in USA is shrinking as Ajay is away from the city most of the time. Even so, if the doctors give us hope and promise, we would love to keep him here. Considering all this, would it be a good idea to take him back to Mumbai where we can keep him at home with required nursing care, along with trying some alternative treatment?'

On the face of his proposal, I instantly said yes because, by that time, I too had become too despondent to carry on with Divyansh in USA. Sighing, I asked him, 'How will we be able to take him to Mumbai in such a condition?' Sushil pensively said, 'If the idea is worth considering, let me work on it.' I knew Sushil: if he took up any project, he would unleash his steadfastness for its success by executing it in the most methodical way.

He first called Dr Reuven Or in Jerusalem to ask if it was a good idea to take Divyansh back to Mumbai and treat him there, considering all aspects. He said, 'That's a wonderful thought. I would prefer taking him to Mumbai for his treatment where I would also like to visit him. But the question is, how will you take him there?' Thanking him for suggestion, Sushil told him, 'If your advice is with me, I will work on it. Unless we think in this direction, we won't find ways to move forward.'

Second, he asked few doctors in the hospital who always empathized with us and treated Divyansh beyond the realm of a patient. They too said that it was the best we could do at that stage. However, they too expressed their apprehension on the logistics of carrying Divyansh to Mumbai.

Third, Sushil thought that before taking Divyansh to Mumbai, there had to be a doctor who should agree to treat him there under his care. He knew Dr C. Deopujari, a neurologist in Mumbai. He texted him a message requesting him for time to talk. Despite being a very busy doctor, Dr Deopujari consented and so Sushil called him. After a detailed discussion, he agreed to treat Divyansh under his care in Mumbai. He sought all his latest medical reports and details of the ongoing treatment. Dr Deopujari talked with straight face and one could misconstrue him as a man with no emotions, but that was not so. Though he maintained his dispassionate composure while talking with Sushil, he couldn't hide the extent of empathy he had for us when he spoke. Before that, he suggested to Sushil to see Dr Rajiv Nanda in Rutgers, New Jersey, a neurologist who happened to be his close friend, for his advice too.

Meanwhile, we actively considered an experimental treatment suggested by a doctor there called stem cell therapy. Sushil met Dr Rajiv Nanda. He saw Divyansh's reports and suggested we take him to Mumbai rather than waste time in USA. When Sushil talked about the prospect of the stem cell therapy, he was quiet for a while. After a short pause, he pensively said:

> Please don't make your son suffer more. I also have a son
> who is a cancer survivor. I know what must be going through
> in your mind. If a child loses his/her father, he is called an
> orphan. If a husband loses his wife, he is called a widower,
> and if a wife loses her husband, she is called a widow. But
> there is no such word for a bereaved parent who loses his
> child. I know this pain as I was very close to reaching this
> stage. Even after understanding all this, both as a human
> being and a doctor, I would advise you to save him from
> unnecessary pain. He came to this world with a purpose.
> As I know, he is exceptionally talented. Please respect his
> dignity. For your son, you are like a God. Do what a God
> is supposed to do at this stage.

After hearing him intently, Sushil thanked him for his timely
advice. In hindsight, meeting Dr Nanda on the advice of Dr
Deopujari was perfectly timed, as it helped us take the decision
to return to Mumbai immediately.

Fourth, and most importantly, we needed to work out the
logistics to take Divyansh back to India. Sushil talked to one airline
through a common contact. They agreed to provide the service.
But it came with a caveat that his travel would be allowed only
if he was accompanied by one qualified nurse or doctor for his
round-the-clock care on the way, and rightly so. We desperately
tried to contact a few Indian nurses in the rehab and elsewhere, but
didn't succeed. For one reason or another, everyone we contacted
to travel with Divyansh expressed their inability. We spent four–
five days looking for one to travel with us, but in vain. We were
dejected and could find no other solution. A mother can take
many avatars for the well-being of her children. So did I. I asked
the nurses there if it was possible for them to train me in the
basics of nursing to enable me to take care of Divyansh during

the travel. They did. They did it by breaking the rules of their profession. They wanted Divyansh to go to his home, and for that, they were willing to do this. Thus, my informal training in nursing care ensued catering to the specific needs of Divyansh. They were more than willing to prepare me for his safe travel. In no time, I picked up the skill with the hands-on guidance given by them.

Sushil had a close friend in Mumbai, a doctor, with whom he discussed his immediate problems and sought guidance from. It is said that when you resolutely try to do something, you will surely find some ways to accomplish that. Unless you conceptualize it and try, there is no way you can achieve anything in your life. Sushil was trying hard to take Divyansh to Mumbai. The Mumbai-based doctor Sushil had contacted was a noble soul. To our huge relief, he offered his own services to facilitate Divyansh's safe journey to Mumbai. He said that he would be with us in the next seven days.

We were already in the second week of July. We planned to return on 21 July. Mridul called us from Dubai informing us that he had taken a leave of 10 days from his office to visit us. He didn't know about our impending plan to return to Mumbai. When I heard about it, I felt that perhaps he was late in visiting his brother now. I doubted if Divyansh would feel his presence at all. I was mindful of Mridul's moral crisis in not having been able to make it there when he was actually required due to his personal and official preoccupations. I thought he should not come now when we planned to return to Mumbai. Nevertheless, I left it to his wisdom. I texted him a message: 'Mridul, it seems you are late now. Perhaps, Divyansh doesn't need you anymore. I feel if you have decided to come, it would only for your own moral redemption. And yes, Sushil would be happy to see you by his side. He always missed you whenever the going was tough for him.' I must admit, Mridul replied to my message with grace and politeness. He was coming in the next two days.

Ajay returned mid-July from his long business visit. When Sushil broke the news of taking Divyansh back to Mumbai, he was astonished and expressed his concern regarding how all this would be possible. We discussed in detail the pros and cons of continuing treatment in USA and convinced him that the cons outweighed the pros. After all, he had been our solid support system, especially for Divyansh, in New Jersey. It was our moral duty to take his consent before going ahead with our decision. Deep in my heart, I still feel for him as he genuinely wanted Divyansh to shine in his life and did everything for him selflessly. Now, as we planned to leave, it must have been his personal loss. His ever-growing affinity for Divyansh got a rude jolt. How deeply Divyansh and he had woven relationship was unfathomable. Perhaps Ajay was another dot that Divyansh's life thread tried to join. Ajay, as I understood him, was an emotionally robust person. His emotions were best reflected through his deeds. It seemed his connection was the best with Divyansh as long as he gave him hope, as long as he rose to Ajay's expectations.

Mridul joined us five days before our departure to Mumbai. Sushil's tired spirit was lifted when Mridul hugged him on his arrival. As long as he was with us, his pain or inability of not making it earlier was palpable on his face. When Harold worked with Divyansh and taught me his unorthodox customized therapy for him before we left, I found Mridul sincerely involved in understanding the finer tricks.

As I packed our bags to leave USA for good, my heart was palpitating. I was transported to last August, when we were at Mumbai airport leaving for New Jersey for Divyansh's admission in FDU. How happy Divyansh was! How happy we were! How happy my parents were! I had never expected to return with Divyansh like this. It seemed life played its choicest and most cruel joke with us. I was sulking. My heart broke a thousand times while I was packing Divyansh's ensemble of T-shirts and shoes into the bag. I almost fainted as I tried to adjust the black suit in the upper flap of the suitcase, which Divyansh had worn on his college visit to the UN office, from where he had sent his proud selfie. I still hoped Divyansh would need it in Mumbai.

We were to leave the rehab by early evening on 21 July. Nurses close to Divyansh and me came one by one, compromising their duties to ensure I took all articles for his medical needs during travel. Some of them broke the rules and secretly gave me a lot of stuff that Divyansh would require. Their eyes were moist but not for themselves. They were for us. They passionately felt that Divyansh should go home. Rehab was not the place for him to live. They also felt that I needed to be united with my family. When they secretly handed over stuff to me, it was soaked with their tears, perhaps to secure Divyansh from any untoward events on the way.

As we left the rehab, all occupants came out to bid us goodbye. Their eyes were moist. I couldn't spot Malina amongst them. As the car started moving, my searching eyes found her standing under the same banyan tree with teary eyes. Perhaps she could not muster the courage to give me farewell hug, as it would have broken her. And yes, this time, I didn't see a cigarette in her hand.

Ajay and Kavita accompanied us to the airport to see us off. Kavita hugged me as we were ready to begin immigration formalities. I too reciprocated and resolved to forgive her for all that she did to us, knowingly or unknowingly.

When the flight took off, it seemed like I was returning after a failed mission.

But was it really a failed mission in the context of the purpose of Divyansh's soul? I began to understand that the purpose of the human body and that of its soul are not the same.

24

FOR THE BALL IS IN YOUR COURT, THE BUCK STOPS WITH YOU

Each one of us is a soul 'system' with a 'thermal equilibrant', called vibes. Now, these vibes take an inherent derivation from the uniqueness that is our nature—a singularity that has no duplicate in the universe. Based on the type of vibes, we people interact and co-exist with each other. The level of equilibrium that we share with another person unfailingly determines what kind of social relations we are going to have. A consonance of vibes, and there is a bonding between people.

—Divyansh, 'Thermodynamics of Life', *Mindcast*

Divyansh's return to Mumbai from USA seemed to be a divine contemplation to complete the journey of his soul. I recalled how teary we were when his neuro-oncologist, Dr Sam, in December last year, had dispassionately told us he would not survive more than two months. The outer limit of his lifeline drawn by him had expired way back. And that's why I was driven to realize that a doctor's assessment of the medical condition of his patients remains within the confines of the human anatomy. Divyansh was relatively better than he was in December–January, when we left the shores of USA. It seemed he had to touch the lives of more people. It also seemed that there were other souls too, who were perhaps waiting to be touched by his.

The aura of Divyansh's face was diminishing with time in USA. To my amazement, it returned when we landed in Mumbai. His face began to glow as if his immediate past was just history. A doctor in Bombay Hospital even remarked that his composed countenance didn't suggest that he was suffering from an acute medical condition. The remark lifted my spirits. I sensed that his soul was trying to stretch one more time to lift me from the abyss of agony.

> When the storm comes,
> Or when harm sways our way,
> I will be the canopy,
> That shades you from this grey.

> ('The Tree of Purity')

From the time of Divyansh's admission to Bombay Hospital after coming back from USA, Dr Deopujari meticulously devised his treatment plan, after examining all his latest reports, by putting the right people on the right job. True to his nature, he threw a word of caution to us about the limitations of medical science considering the complexity of Divyansh's medical problems, adding that from here on, his condition would only worsen. And then, I saw Divyansh's glowing and captivating face, around which the nurses and other paramedics loved to flock. Without paying too much heed to Dr Deopujari's comments, I resolved to take one day at a time.

Dr Deopujari had engaged for Divyansh's care Ms Roshan Vania, a renowned neuro-therapist of the hospital. Ms Vania, an octogenarian, was a short Parsi lady, whose wrinkled face displayed her vast experience in the profession. She looked frail at first sight. But when she shook my hand with her firm grip, I immediately realized that it was a therapist's grip which didn't lose its tautness with age. At her age, her assistants intently followed her with great admiration and utmost respect. While in USA, I wondered about the kind of therapists Divyansh would get in India. I thought their medical science and other allied services like neuro-physiotherapy were the best in the world. In fact, I heard the term neuro-therapist for the first time in USA. I wondered if I would find a comparable one, if not better, in Mumbai. I realized how wrong I was after meeting Ms Vania and her team. I began to be healed by the calmness of the words she spoke. True to the ethos of Zoroastrianism, she tried to sensitize me with the power of prayer. Apart from herself, she released five powerful souls from her quiver, like five fingers of a palm waiting to hold Divyansh in their grip. Yes, their souls were waiting to be touched by Divyansh's. They were Pallavi, Abhinav, Zainab, Fatema and Mansi, whose services were diligently planned by Ms Vania for Divyansh's well-being at home after his discharge from the hospital on 5 August.

Divyansh came back home after a year, his soul much enriched and perhaps content for its existential meaning after his American sojourn. He didn't stay in the room he had before his travel to USA. That was usually his study room at home. He had graduated by then in his life. The guest room in our home was better equipped to cater to his day-to-day needs. His entry into the guest room was seemingly symbolic and divinely guided.

Our family was finally reunited. Ananya got her brother along with the ball to play 'Catch–Catch'. The semblance of our family life seemed to be coming back. Whatever difficulties we were facing, we were still able to give the best to Divyansh. He looked better and was more expressive while trying to extricate himself from his problems. His response to all the five therapists was more than therapeutic.

Pallavi, a neuro-physiotherapist, over a period of time, became Divyansh's soulmate. She was a young girl, newly married to a handsome young man. She looked like a thorough professional to me. But she became like a family member to us and a sister to Divyansh. She not only performed therapy to the best of her ability but also tried everything to pull him out of his deep trance. On the days her sessions were good, she was on top of the world with joy. On the days she felt it was not good, she was sad and dejected. Her affinity for Divyansh grew to an extent that she never missed her sessions with him even a single day. One day, her husband called Sushil to convince her not to come for session as she was sick, but she was hell-bent on visiting Divyansh. She was the one who guided the team of five on what would work for him. She often said that Divyansh was like a star in her eyes, a star which sparkled in the darkness to enlighten her with the wisdom with which he lived. She talked to me after her sessions to know his life's journey. She read his various poems and blogs. Divyansh's inspiration on her was visible. She expressed to me her wish to celebrate her birthday with him. We happily agreed. She openly wished for a gift from me—that Divyansh would wear a red shirt, and so would she. We celebrated her birthday in the way she wished. More than the celebration of her birthday, it was the consonance of vibes between the two souls that I saw. I never noticed when the professional boundary had been left behind by her while working with him.

The tall and handsome Abhinav was barely five years older than Divyansh. He was sharp in his profession, quick to read emerging medical conditions and would accordingly fine-tune his sessions. With time, he too was attracted to Divyansh's soul and attempted everything even beyond the realm of his profession to make him better. He treated him like a younger brother. He once had to go to Amritsar for some personal work. When he returned, he brought a kada for Divyansh to bring good fortune to his life. The extent of his closeness is understood with the text message he once sent Sushil:

We waited for his responses every time, and when that small response appeared, there was a ray of hope, which would get us fired up even more. Yes, we can do it. Yes, we can make him better. This was the time Divyansh became closer, rather I was pulled into his sterling aura (which I would avoid otherwise because it would be unprofessional). I got to hear stories of his struggles, and how each time he evolved through it, came up even stronger. Trust me, it wasn't normal, it wasn't usual. His mom was there as the strongest pillar of support holding the boy, fighting for him; you narrated his childhood stories and this guy would quietly listen to all them, relishing them silently. As the days passed, he was not just a patient. He communicated many things without speaking; it was just a matter of connection. I was so touched by his life that he became a younger sibling to me. His write-ups inspired me, his attitude astonished me, as a person I was deeply influenced by him.

After the sessions, I ensured that he was served with those dishes I would have served my son.

Zainab worked on Divyansh's auditory stimulation. She too was a young girl of Pallavi's age. When she came to see Divyansh at Bombay Hospital, the first thing she did after evaluating him was to read his poem 'Here We Go Again,' when she heard that he wrote poetry. She was so inspired after reading the poem that she took on his case as a challenge to make him better. She saw in him an even bigger fighter to respond to her stimulation. During her regular visits to our home, she often read his poems and blogs and would reflect that Divyansh had an uncanny knack of looking at life and things from different perspectives, some of which were just extraordinary. She often told me after the sessions that he, through body language and eyes, communicated a lot and told her so much. There were times he would not respond. Then she would explain to him her plan, which he would listen to intently. She confessed to me that Divyansh had left a strong mark in her life even without speaking in words.

One good thing Zainab unknowingly did for Divyansh was to bring his music teacher Savio back in his life. She didn't know Savio, though. One day, after the session, she advised to engage a good musician for his auditory and sensory stimulation. Savio instantly flashed in our minds. But we had been completely out of touch for a long time, though Divyansh occasionally interacted with him through text messages from USA. We somehow found his mobile number and requested him to visit Divyansh after narrating his present medical condition. He was not aware of all that had happened. After talking to Zainab, he promised to come in two days. It was such a wonderful and emotional sight to behold when he met Divyansh after such a long period. As soon as Divyansh saw Savio enter his room, guitar strapped to his shoulder, he began connecting with him. It seemed like he wanted to say something to him, but couldn't. He felt dejected and expressed his pain through his facial expression to him. Savio managed to hold in his emotions somehow. And then the saga of the duo, Zainab and Savio, began for Divyansh. Savio would often reflect on the past time spent with Divyansh where he engaged him through intellectual discussion and laughter. He was so moved to see his indefatigable efforts to respond to his sessions with Zainab that he wrote to Sushil one day, 'It was a joy to encourage and inspire his desire to learn the skill of making music his life, and in return, his diligence was very rewarding. Even as he is struggling with the inertia of his health these days, he kept pushing forward and never gave up. His persistence and perseverance will always be inspiration for me. I am glad I am a part of his journey in this endeavour.'

I believed there was something Divyansh had still to share with Savio, which was accomplished when he came back into his life, thanks to Zainab.

The other two physiotherapists, namely, Mansi and Fatema, became Divyansh's soulmates as well as they spent more time with him. Fatema joined us at a later stage, at the direction of Ms Vania, for specialized therapy. She was slightly older than Divyansh. She often told me that she never saw any cases like Divyansh, where a patient rose every time after he fell. She was hopeful that this time too, he would make it. Her motivation from Divyansh's inspirational journey was visible when she worked with him with all the affection at her command. As for Mansi, as Pallavi told me, she, for the first time, breached her professional boundaries in Divyansh's case, and did many things for him that she would perhaps not do for other patients.

By mid-September, Divyansh began showing some signs of recovery. He responded to the therapies and began responding to us emotively and trying to connect as much as possible. Every morning when I woke up, I would think of a better day for my son and hope that he would recover fully someday. The reason for the new-found hope was Divyansh himself, the way he was trying to rise like a phoenix from the ashes one more time. However, by the time I retired for bed at night, I recalled the events of the day, his suffering, his desire to see smiles on my face and so many other things, and I prayed for the end of his ceaseless suffering. And again, the next day I would wake up with a fresh lease on life. I trusted Divyansh's self-belief and my own too, which owed its origin to Divyansh's, and tried to bounce back to begin the day with new vigour.

Two other people were waiting to re-enter Divyansh's life. Raji Madam, his yoga teacher, called me one day wishing to meet him. Even though we had restricted visitors from seeing Divyansh for fear of him catching infections, how could I have said no to her? Though she had a soft and caring heart, she normally didn't reflect her emotional side. That's how she was. When she saw Divyansh after more than a year that day, he connected with her; she couldn't stop her emotions flowing from her eyes. She remained with him for some time and gave her yogic talk to invoke his spirit; all the while Divyansh listened to her with great respect. Every time Raji Madam addressed him as Chhota Hanuman, his facial expression changed, as if he too wanted to say something. She had often told Divyansh in his heydays that his name and conduct reminded her of a divine soul. She fondly remembered her conversations with him on subjects ranging from philosophy, general psychology and various other topics related to the cosmos. She had once told us, 'His eyes were always sparkling and one could clearly notice the thirst for acquiring knowledge about every little thing in the world. This greatest quality was loving and doting on the people close to him. Unconditional was his affection. His mother doted on him, but his love for his mother and his only sister was something unparalleled. My words will fall short to narrate his love for his mother; none of my drawn pictures can explain.'

Yes, the consonance of their soulful vibes was apparent even now as Divyansh communicated with her non-verbally.

Ahreman napak; ahreman khak shaved, ahreman dur shaved, ahreman dafe shaved, ahreman shekasteh shaved, ahreman halak shaved.

Ms Rati Wadia, Divyansh's ex-English teacher, began visiting him twice a week. The first thing she did was take a clean white handkerchief and pass it over him from head to toe without touching him, while repeating the above words from their holy book Avesta. It means: let all negativities, satanic and evil, which cause ailments, be expelled from his body and let his body welcome all positivity. When she repeated these holy words, she visualized all his ailments disappearing. The resolve to bring about positive change in Divyansh was apparent from her serene face. After the prayer, she would read out Divyansh's poem in our presence to invoke in the underlying spirit with which he had written them. As long as she remained with him, I would observe her soothing effect on him. Here, too, the consonance of vibes of two powerful souls was conspicuous by the magical effect it created.

I always wondered about Divyansh's divine connection with Rati Wadia. How could she become so close to her student when she hardly taught him for two months? I remembered that when Divyansh returned from Israel after transplantation, he had brought her a thoughtful souvenir, a silver-cased Torah, holy book of the Jews, considering her interest in reading and collecting the holy books of other religions. He knew in those two months that this was the only holy book she didn't have. In those two months, he also knew that the great thespian Dilip Kumar was her heartthrob. That's why he gifted her Dilip Kumar's biography on her birthday. A teacher of Rati Wadia's stature is always a teacher, no matter how far her students move on in their lives.

Ananya was due to appear for her Class 10 board examination early the next year. Divyansh often expressed his pain at not being able to help her in studies in the manner he wished. At our urging, it became Ananya's daily chore to narrate to him how her preparations were going on and how best her studies were being taken care of by her teachers and Papa. A distinct sigh would invariably appear from him every time Ananya spoke to him about her progress. There were times when Sushil taught her in Divyansh's room when he was awake, just to assuage him that everything on the study front was fine. This is also a fact that despite all these daily challenges going on at home, we ensured her studies proceeded without much disturbance. One should strike a chord of normalcy in whatever adverse situation one is, only then such adverse situations will render you to lead at least a semblance of a normal life. I learnt this maxim of life from Divyansh time and again.

Towards mid-October, Divyansh's condition began deteriorating acutely without any visible trigger. The attending doctors could not figure out any immediate reason. However, the condition was such that it required ICU care in the hospital. We tried to avoid his hospitalization by convincing doctors to manage him from home. However, we realized our folly a few days later. Divyansh was admitted to the ICU of Bombay Hospital on 25 October 2018. His blood pressure was dipping. With the intervention of a novel IV drug, they were able to stabilize his blood pressure. The doctors categorically told Sushil that it was very difficult to pull him back from the condition he was in. It was a question of a few days only. We were still holding on to our spirit.

25

I MARCH FORWARD, WITH A STRONG SPIRIT, WITH ALL GUNS BLAZING

D r Vibhor, the attending neurologist, came to visit Divyansh one day. After he examined him, he called me to the nursing station and told me about his precarious medical condition. He asked me to decide if I intended to keep him in hospital or take him home for his comfortable last few days. Sushil was not with me then; he was at his office. There were about five nurses listening to the doctor. I heard him quietly, and handed him Divyansh's poem 'Here We Go Again' to read and, through it, I succinctly apprised him of our, and more importantly, Divyansh's valiant spirit. Dr Vibhor was so moved after reading the poem that he could hardly control his eyes turning teary. I asked him to advise me after reading the poem what I should do. He did not say much. Later, I was told, he proudly gave this poem to many people to read to let them know about the determination of his patient and his family, and decided to continue his treatment at the hospital under his able care.

It was Diwali on 7 November. Divyansh was on the brink of his life in the hospital. We didn't allow the true spirit of this festival to be missed even on that day. We lit candles outside the ICU in festive fervour. We saw the visage of Divyansh's soul in the dazzle of flames of the candles as they danced with every gentle blow of air caressing their surface. The luminance of the flames spread the spirit of his soul far and wide. The flames were celebrating the triumph of Divyansh's soul over the likely end of his body's journey.

Fatema and Ms Vania gave me moral support in a big way during this period too. They visited Divyansh every day and kept showing me the light of hope. I was, by then, mentally ready to face any eventuality. Sometimes the situation of hopelessness ironically results in incognizant toughness in us, with which we try to learn to live with the problems on hand. This incognizant toughness made my resolve even stronger to observe the Chhath fast, beginning on 13 November, even though Divyansh was battling for his life in the ICU. Chhath, as the years passed, no longer remained a festival for me. It was a matter of pride. It instilled in me a unique feeling of completeness in my womanhood and a feeling of purity. I had been keeping Chhath for the last eight years. This year, I was determined to do it for the completeness of my motherhood for Divyansh. If the doctors had left everything to Divyansh's body to take its course, I, on the other hand, felt his life was under the care of his mighty soul and my motherhood. Divyansh's soul was doing its part. My motherhood had to do its part to bring about the consonance of vibes Divyansh talked about in his blog, 'Thermodynamics of Life'.

Sushil was apprehensive about my plan to go ahead with Chhath. At the end of the day, though Divyansh was being adequately taken care of by nurses and doctors, we were supposed to be in the ICU round the clock. If life gives you opportunities, grab it. If it throws challenges at you, face them with all the might at your command. I was ready to face it. I fasted the whole day while being with Divyansh in the ICU. We went to the Girgaum Chowpatty in the evening to offer my obeisance to the Sun God. But this time, while offering Argha to him, I didn't wish for anything. There was no hope I could get a boon from him. Time forced me to worship on this Chhath with complete detachment. I was doing this only for myself and for Divyansh. I was propitiating that part of Goddess Parvati in me that Divyansh had visualized I was bestowed with when he was born to me. After the evening worship, I came back to the ICU with the divinity that motherhood had brought about in me. The next morning, too, after offering Argha to the Sun God, I came back to the hospital to take care of Divyansh. While I sat by his side holding his hand, I thought how happy Divyansh would have been to know I could do Chhath even this time around.

As we approached the end of November, Divyansh was able to sustain his blood pressure without the intervention of the novel drug. Gradually, the doctor weaned him off that drug. The doctors were clueless. When he was admitted a month back, they had told us his chances of survival were bleak. It seemed the tides were turning in his favour. I was not expecting any miracle. Yet, I was healing as I saw Divyansh fighting to come back. And then, an unanticipated event took place. Pain no more surprised us. Happiness did.

As the doctors planned to discharge Divyansh in the beginning of December, Sushil casually asked them to do a scan of his brain if they thought it advisable, just to ascertain how much it had worsened. The doctor politely obliged us and recommended a CT scan, knowing fully well that it was a sheer waste of money. The scan result came by evening to the nurses' station of the ICU. The resident doctors on duty whispered among themselves to ensure we didn't get to listen to what they were talking about. I thought they were hiding the reports from us to save us from anxiety. When Sushil emphatically asked them to let us know the report, one of them said that some miraculous changes had been noticed in the brain as per the scan. They waited for a senior doctor to brief us about it. The doctor came in the late evening and said that the reports suggested significant improvement in the brain, much to their surprise. Initially, he thought that this report was mixed up with some other patient's, but after ascertaining from the lab, he confirmed that it was Divyansh's report. Divyansh's brain scan had been consistently showing a deteriorating picture since last September. There was no occasion it had ever shown any improvement. Since he was admitted to the hospital this time, he had not been given any new medicine that may have worked magically. The doctors didn't have any answer to the magical change happening. While the news brought us much needed jubilance, all the while I thought it was some unfinished work which Divyansh's soul had yet to complete, which perhaps resulted in the improvement in his brain condition. His soul, it seemed, rekindled the fire in him again. With this feel-good factor, the doctor was more than happy to discharge him on 5 December for continued home care.

Divyansh began showing steady progress in the next two months. He tried to interact more emotionally, responded to the therapies and listened to the music we often played. We never forgot to play Niladri Kumar's 'Plucked' every day, one of his favourites. Apart from regular therapy, Rati Wadia's regular visits became a family feature for us. All this resulted in rekindling new hope in him. I took baby steps in dreaming for Divyansh again. Being able to hope, from a situation of hopelessness, can be very empowering, and I began noticing it in me. I would sit by his side holding his hand tightly the whole day. It was just to reassure him and me that we would stand with each other, no matter what the situation.

Divyansh's twenty-second birthday was on 27 January 2019. I figured out from his vibes that he didn't want any formal celebration on this day. What a contrast I was seeing in him! There were days in his early life when he meticulously planned his birthday and ensured his choicest gift from us. Likewise, with equal fervour, he did the same when we celebrated our birthdays or wedding anniversary. It seemed that he now found it mundane to celebrate his twenty-second, perhaps the last one: he knew, we didn't. The transformation I was witnessing in him shook me completely. Even though I myself didn't want to celebrate his birthday this time, the subtle message coming from his side unnerved me. But forget us; we were literally served a writ by his therapists to celebrate his day in a big way. We had to give in and allowed them to celebrate in whatever way they wanted. After all, Divyansh's soul belonged to them equally. However, at no stage did I find Divyansh absorbed in their celebration. He was lost somewhere, completely withdrawn.

Time was ticking away. Ananya's board exams started in the third week of February. She would come back from the exam and sit with us in Divyansh's room, discussing how well she had performed. While we discussed her papers, he would look affectionately at her. Ananya too sensed how relieving it was for Divyansh when she said she had done well in the exams. Every time she left home for the examination centre, she took his blessings. In what way Divyansh blessed her, only Ananya and he knew. The profoundness of non-verbal communication was optimum when I saw the sublime effect of their interactions. In the first week of March, I found Divyansh in distress again, warranting frequent visits from his doctors. His condition deteriorated fast in the next few days, yet he held on to his nerves to avoid hospitalization. He was waiting for something to happen before losing control on his cognition. Ananya's examination was to end on 19 March. The day her exams got over and we discussed her performance in Divyansh's presence, I saw him heave a big sigh of relief and then he gradually began sinking. He had painfully waited for this day to ensure her hassle-free completion of exams from his side. He never wanted her to suffer because of his own medical condition. By that evening, his condition became so bad that he had to be hospitalized.

Divyansh was in the ICU. Sushil and I were discussing if it was a coincidence that Ananya's completion of examination and

Divyansh's hospitalization happened just one after the other. We would never know for sure the answer to this question, but we could feel it. This time his hospitalization was not for long. He was discharged in seven days. However, his overall condition at the time of discharge was not good. But it was deemed appropriate to take care of him in the home set-up.

Divyansh's condition never improved after that. It went steadily downhill. I spent entire days in his room holding his hand, subconsciously infusing him with all my motherly resolve, trying to satiate him with the tender touch he always craved. I talked about his early childhood, his school days, his friends, his poems and what not. I consciously tried to rewind his whole life journey in my trembling voice. Wherever I fumbled while doing so, I felt him hold my hand more tightly, signalling his support yet another time for me to lean on. It seemed he wanted to listen more from me.

Divyansh's condition continued worsening. He was admitted to the hospital on 18 April for difficulty in breathing. A quick brain scan revealed impairment of that area of the brain that controlled involuntary breathing and other vitals of the body. He was on life support now. The doctors said that it was a matter of only a few more days. This time I didn't question their assessment. My motherly instinct was enough to indicate that he was on his way to complete his last circumambulation. But the aura of his face spoke differently. I remained seated by his side, holding his hand all day to continue giving him my tender touch. Looking at his face, a person could never imagine his condition was so acute. Ms Roshan Vania came to visit him every day. While he lay quietly on life support, after meeting him one day, she remarked that she had seen a big halo on his forehead and that he seemed to reflect the Dalai Lama. She, with complete poise, whispered to me in her trembling voice, 'I am secretly telling you, Divyansh is with God now.'

Till then, his other vitals were functioning, though at abnormal levels. Ms Rati Wadia, true to her nature, came to the hospital daily to offer prayers for him. It was 1 May. Ms Wadia reached the hospital at 5 p.m. I was getting a push from within. After she finished her prayers, I requested her to read aloud Divyansh's poem 'Catharsis'. She was just waiting for this opportunity, and I believe she was guided by her own instinct as well.

Ms Wadia began reading the poem. Then, she called Sushil and again read out the poem. It seemed Divyansh was driving us to do something which he would have liked to do.

> Let's see what You "have in store" for me
> For the ball is in Your court,
> The Buck is on You,
> As I march forward, with a strong spirit,
> And with all guns blazing.

Ms Wadia didn't stop. At my request, she called all the nurses and doctors in the ICU and asked them to listen to her reflections about Divyansh.

Was it Divyansh's wish to complete his last circumambulation with his paraph?

The nurses and the doctors on duty in the ICU quietly obliged. Ms Wadia then narrated Divyansh's virtues and her experience with him after long association. Every person became numb. She then read out 'Catharsis' again. As she was reading his poem, everyone present there had tears in their eyes. But Divyansh was gazing at the proceedings with closed eyes, with utmost calm and a revitalized aura. It appeared as if he wanted someone to read out his communication with God through this poem before he finally went into his lap. He wanted him to know that he was soon coming to him. Divyansh had started his medical journey from Bombay Hospital in December 2009 and was going to complete it here itself in 2019. All his life, whatever he wanted to achieve or get, he tried to grab it with all his means. Once he decided to leave something, he did that without any qualms. It seemed his soul had now decided to leave his body for its salvation. True to his nature, he was still well poised, reflecting a shining aura from his face while his soul was completing its journey.

The next morning, 2 May 2019, Divyansh's soul left his body. The divine motherhood, which he had brought into my soul through his birth, perhaps also left me along with him.

Yes, Divyansh's visit to earth for 22 years was not long, but it was definitely big. It encapsulated all the karmas and the dharmas of a life cycle.

On the fourth day after he moved to a different world, we organized a prayer meeting for Divyansh, where several people came to offer their condolences. I was completely shaken by the very idea of attending a prayer meeting for my son. I had never attended any such prayer meeting in the past. I never thought a day would come in my life where I would have to attend my son's prayer meeting. As long as I was there, I was numb. It seemed like my body was forcibly kept there. The well of my tears had dried up by then. While the bhajan choir was singing, Ms Wadia requested Sushil to allow her to speak to the guests about Divyansh from the dais. Reluctantly, Sushil nodded, and the bhajan was stopped for a while. She went up to the dais, sat on a chair and began speaking about Divyansh, his life journey, his literary excellence and people of all religions whose lives he had touched in his short yet meaningful life. She completed her speech on a personal note of her association with him and how her own life at her age was impacted by him. And then, she read out his poem, 'Catharsis'. The rendition of the poem was so powerful that everyone present there became teary.

On the way back home after the prayer meeting, ironically, I felt relieved. I felt like I had attended an award function for my son, thanks to Ms Wadia, the teacher, who introduced her student to the audience in a way befitting his deeds. Most of those who had come for the prayer knew Divyansh as our son. Ms Wadia's emotional speech and recitation of his poem gave him a crystal clear and distinct identity in their eyes, one he would be known for, independent of us.

Months later, Ananya and I went to Kemps Corner in Mumbai to buy something. It was monsoon time and that day, it was raining incessantly. I carried an umbrella for any exigency. It happened to be a Divyansh's umbrella which he had used during his college days in USA, and it was my treasured possession. When I finished my shopping, an impoverished mother with her two children, one on her hips and the other one holding her finger, came to me begging for money. I gave her some money. But that mother also begged for an umbrella for the safety of her children in the heavy rains. Without thinking much, I parted ways with my treasured possession. I gave Divyansh's umbrella to another mother to protect her Divyansh. I came back home with my eyes moist.

꧁꧂

26

THE FATHER SPEAKS...

HOLY PEOPLE IN A HOLY LAND

Divyansh had written a blog titled 'A World without Religion':

> Can't we live and thrive in a world devoid of religion? A world where humanity, kindness, unity, love, righteousness and dignity are the values that form the alternative to Religion.

I experienced this in the holy land of Israel where three religions, namely, Judaism, Islam and Christianity, co-exist in an uncharacteristic way. However, all three religions lose their central characters and fuse to become one common religion when it comes to serving mankind.

The decision to visit Jerusalem for Divyansh's treatment was taken all of a sudden in the month of March 2015. Considering his medical condition and the promise of a sustainable cure that the Holy Land provided him, we began our journey to Jerusalem on 29 March. The people we came across there and who lent their helping hands when it mattered the most, gave me an insight that this Holy Land was truly inhabited by holy people. In order to foster belief in a pan-world religion of humanity as envisaged by Divyansh, such people need to be remembered, written and discussed far and wide.

Dr Reuven Or: Toda Raba

6 February 2015

After a brief respite, the days of agony seemed to have begun again. I was sitting in an isolated corner of the car park of Bombay Hospital in complete despair. Had it returned again? If yes, what would I do now? How would I face him when the likely news was broken to Divyansh? All of a sudden, a thought came to my mind. Enough is enough. If that happens again, I will now change the approach. A glimmer of hope set in me. Many a time, the subconscious mind helps guide the conscious mind when one is clueless about one's next move. It controls all the vital processes of our body and knows the answer to each problem. There was something in-situ at a subconscious level which was now readying me to face a new daunting task ahead with new hope. Dr Reuven Or was the reason for this hope.

We reached Jerusalem on 30 March 2015. After checking into the apartment, we proceeded to the Hadassah Hospital straightway, where Dr Or worked. The moment we stepped onto the third floor where his office was located, I saw a tall, light-eyed man, 6 feet plus, wearing a black kippah on his head, approaching us briskly.

'Hello, Mr Poddar and Divyansh. Welcome to the holy land of Jerusalem. I am Dr Reuven Or. I have heard a lot about your son, and we together will do everything for him to ameliorate him from his nagging medical problem,' he said and hugged Divyansh and then me.

'Dr Reuven, we have come here with a lot of hope. Please treat my son in the best possible manner,' I said with a heavy heart.

'Don't worry, I will not only treat your son but also pray for him in our synagogue,' was his reply. He then guided me through the initial formalities of the hospital. With his very first look and interaction, Dr Reuven Or seemed more of an angel than a doctor. It felt like we had reached the right person. I wondered if a doctor could be like him.

Dr Reuven Or was a semi-orthodox Jew whose philosophy of treating his patients was on a different paradigm. He maintained that treating a patient was nothing but serving humanity, and service to humanity has to be godly. Yes, it seemed the healing touch had already begun before the actual treatment could start. In the beginning, since most of the establishments in Israel were closed in lieu of the Passover festival, he suggested that we should visit the important places in Israel to absorb the spirit of the Holy Land. Apparently, his approach to treating his patients was holistic, which transcended the usual boundaries of medical science. Whenever Divyansh visited any important places in Jerusalem and narrated his experience to him, he felt excited to listen to his narration. He often said, 'Let me do my part and you do your part of keeping yourself in the right spirit. If you need any help in doing your part, please do not hesitate to call me.' We had never had the experience of dealing with a doctor who commanded such colossal stature and pervaded the soul of patients and their caregivers so deeply.

In our initial days, we had lot of questions relating to the procedure of transplantation. He always encouraged us to raise those questions by saying, 'Divyansh, that's an intelligent question.' And then he would answer all our concerns. He also made it a point to ask about the well-being of our family back in Mumbai at the end of each meeting. The extent of his empathy for us was such that he often, without my knowledge, asked for a discount in various departments of the hospital in order to provide us some financial relief. I never knew why he did this as our relationship didn't go too far back.

Medically, the transplantation under his care was completed in textbook style. During our hospital stay, we saw that he commanded huge respect not only from doctors, but also from all the paramedics and other support staff. He was very pleased with Divyansh's post-transplantation progress and the way he cooperated in following all medical advice with a smile on his face. His special love and care for Divyansh was discernible. When Divyansh was recovering in the hospital after the procedure, he resumed his studies for Class 12 exams that he had to miss earlier that year. This pleased Dr Or very much. He remarked, 'Divyansh, it is heavenly to see you studying for exams in the hospital—thus, you have bridged the gap between the hospital and home.' To this, Divyansh politely replied, 'Doctor, you have brought my home to your hospital. Let me do my part in my new home.' Such was the camaraderie between Dr Reuven and Divyansh.

After discharge from the hospital, when we were in the apartment, Dr Or invariably called us to follow-up on Divyansh's progress. There were times when I was forced to call him from our apartment at midnight to take his advice. He picked up every call of mine without fail, offered all assistance and promised to visit our apartment if the need arose. I never realized that medical service could be so godly.

In mid-August, two months after the transplantation, when we had gone to see him for Divyansh's periodical follow-up, I asked Dr Or to give me some time after he was through with the check-up. Some thoughts had been going on in my mind for the past few days which I wanted to share with him and take his advice.

'Dr Or, it's been almost six months since we came here. Divyansh is staying here only for the follow-up. My wife and daughter are in Mumbai. I think in his recovery phase post transplantation, he would require the care of his mother as well, apart from the excellent medical care you are providing. Do you suggest planning our trip to Mumbai now? Is it medically advisable?' I hesitatingly asked Dr Or.

'Oh! Why not! You can do that. Please let me know the doctor under whose care you wish to put him for follow-ups in Mumbai.

I will collaborate with him on phone as well as via mail. I think that's a good idea. But before that, allow me to take you all for a family dinner if you don't mind,' Dr Or gave his assuring reply.

It was humbling for us to see a doctor in an alien country taking us for a family dinner. Respecting his sentiment, we agreed, and I asked him to give me the address we were supposed to reach. He said he would come to our apartment to pick us up.

1 September 2015

Divyansh, after breakfast, was in a thoughtful mood. When I enquired what he was thinking about, he said, 'Papa, I am thinking of writing a letter to Dr Or to express my gratitude to him for all that he has done for me. It's not a usual doctor–patient relationship. I will hand over the letter to him when we meet today evening for dinner. That's my way of conveying Toda Raba to him.'

I was enthused to feel his manner of saying thanks.

Dr Or and his wife Hani came to pick us up at the appointed time in the evening, and took us to an open-air restaurant outside the city. We enjoyed the food and had lot of informal conversations. Divyansh then requested them to allow him to read his letter to Dr Or before giving it to him.

Here goes his Toda Raba letter:

Whoever saves one life saves the world entire.

—Itzhak Stern, *Schindler's List*

Very profound quote. Found it really apt to word my gratitude for you in one line. Yes, Doctor. You have actually saved my life, and also of those who are part of my world— the lives of my father, mother, sister and my closest family.

If you look at the main poster of the movie *Schindler's*

List, it portrays a larger hand from above holding a smaller, helpless hand below in its clutch. Nothing is a more appropriate description of you, my doctor, and I, coming to you as a helpless patient. Honestly, when my leukaemia relapsed for the second time, all of us could feel nothing but despair around us, especially myself. It was then that Dr Archana mentioned BMT along with your name. That was a ray of hope. As God willed, I was fortunate, by his design, to come to perhaps one of the holiest cities in the world for my treatment. Dr Archana had also told us her description of you, 'The first time we saw him, 6 feet plus, and light eyed, it was as if he was the angel God sent to cure my son.' Well, could not have been more true. The vibes and positive energy you exude, the personal attention to every want of your patient, that radiant smile, and most importantly, your attitude that says to a patient, 'Don't worry. Everything is alright' truly makes you, at least for me, as someone from heaven.

Thank you, Doctor Reuven Or, for lifting me with your firm grasp from a six-year-long arduous, leukaemic journey. That's all I can say, along with one more thing. May God really bless you.

Always bowed in gratitude,

1 September 2015   Divyansh Atman

Dr Or and Hani were speechless after Divyansh read out his letter. Controlling his emotions, Dr Or only said that this was one of the most precious gifts he had ever received from his patients. He stood up and gave a return Toda Raba to Divyansh with a tight hug.

I thought nothing could have been a more befitting way to end our long association with Dr Or before we left the Holy Land.

But I was wrong.

This letter actually laid the foundation stone for a long-standing relation with him, perhaps stronger than ever before.

Six months after transplantation, Divyansh developed some complications. We went back to see Dr Or after Divyansh finished his Class 12 exams. Considering the nature of the complications, Dr Or prescribed a medicine which was too costly and not even available in Israel. It brings tears to my eyes to write that he arranged for this medicine not once, but twice, from Germany, free of cost, for Divyansh, using his good relations with the pharmaceutical company. Dr Or must have seen thousands of patients in his lifetime, but the level of his relationship with Divyansh spoke something else. There was a definite divinity attached to this which was beyond my comprehension.

We returned to Mumbai after the new treatment from Israel. A year later, as luck would have it, Divyansh had another relapse. With no more treatment options available either in India or Israel, Dr Or advised me to take Divyansh to USA for a treatment which was then in trial stage. Dr Or continued to remain in touch with the doctor in USA treating Divyansh. As he was recovering post treatment there, Divyansh took admission in a university in New Jersey to pursue his dream of becoming a computer engineer. We were happy. Dr Or was happy.

But our joy didn't last long. Divyansh finally relapsed for the last time. Doctors tried hard, first in USA and later, in Mumbai, unsuccessfully. Divyansh's soul had decided to move to a better place.

Dr Or wrote to me:

Dear Family Poddar,

On behalf of myself and Hani, including the bone marrow transplant team, I would like to share with you the great loss of your beloved son.

Divyansh's special personality and wisdom had a deep impression on our thoughts and hearts.

I was impressed with him from the very first moment

of our meeting. The very first look of his suggested that he was a very mature and a brave person and was willing to do everything to overcome the disease. Since then he has been my role model. He always evoked positivity towards the treatment, the medicines he was subjected to and the essence of life. I must say, he was coping with the disease spiritually, a trait which is rarely seen in other patients. He was a young man, still in his teens, but spoke like a mature adult and a realistic person having immense faith in the science of medicine. His soul was very special. As doctors, we study and investigate the anatomy of the human body. But we don't know how to investigate the anatomy of the soul. He was an example for me and the entire team of doctors and nurses of the bone marrow department of the hospital. He always cared for others. He was doing everything for himself and his family. To me, he was a holy soul. Everything he said came from his heart. In Hebrew, there is a saying which means that some people have a smart brain–heart connection. Divyansh was one such person. He was like a prophet in the Bible.

I think Divyansh's unique personality was built up by his family. I think what his parents did for him, we rarely see often. In my 40 years of experience in dealing with cancer patients, I have not come across such [parents who were] ready to cross any limit to treat their son. Divyansh is, therefore, a fruit of his parents. Unfortunate events like death of their son didn't stop them from loving Divyansh's friends and persons like us.

We hope to see you in the near future so we can express together our mutual love for Divyansh.

Always yours,
Reuven

Dr Or and my family are still in touch. He is still holding us with his larger hand from above as Divyansh had felt and expressed.

Now is my time to say Toda Raba to Dr Or as I write this memoir for him.

◆

Ethereal Leuma and Her Khamsa

Towards the end of our first visit to Jerusalem, sometime in the third week of July 2015, I got an unexpected call from an old lady named Leuma. She introduced herself in a soft voice and said that she was a friend of Dr Archana, our friend in Mumbai. She apparently was concerned on hearing what Divyansh was going through in Jerusalem. She politely invited us to her home in a nearby neighbourhood on the following Sabbath. When I asked for her address, she said that her husband Gideon would fetch us from our apartment. Then, I recalled that Dr Archana had talked about her when we were leaving for Jerusalem. Though invites like this used to be showered on us from our new-found friends there, some of who were Jews, I was quite reticent to accept this invitation thinking Leuma must be an old lady who I didn't wish to overburden with hosting a dinner for us. What moved me and changed my decision was the softness and calmness of her voice which seemed to have come straight from her heart and reached us with the same intensity.

Leuma Lerman was a charming old lady of about 80 years of age. The old saying that age is just a number was aptly applied in her case. Shoulder length, well-trimmed grey hair and dressed for the occasion, she was immaculate to the core. When she smiled, the wrinkles on her face also smiled with the same amplitude. Her big light eyes spoke more than her mouth. Her husband, Gideon, was a tall man who could easily beat any youngster with the energy levels he possessed. Her two daughters, Irit and Orna, exuded the effervescent persona of their mother. She had special fetish for owls. A glass cabinet in her living room displayed a huge collection of owls of all hues and sizes, which were sourced from various countries as she told me.

When Divyansh and I reached her home, she was waiting for us at the door. She hugged Divyansh and planted a motherly kiss on his cheeks and then she turned to me and greeted me with 'Sabbath Shalom', followed by the same enticing hug and a motherly kiss. I didn't know that the warmth of a very first meeting with a stranger could be so divine. In a few interactions with Divyansh, she developed a tremendous liking for him. Divyansh was equally charmed by her bountiful affection, which instantly made him talk freely to her. At no stage did it appear that we were meeting for the first time. The food spread on the dining table was lavish, all cooked by her, of course, with the help of her soulmate Gideon. She had an eclectic taste in food. We savoured the food; our hosts touched our souls more than the gastronomical delights. It was a perfect retreat from an otherwise monotonous life there. What I liked the most about Leuma was her curiosity and inquisitiveness to understand our cultural values, but at the same time, not being too verbose about hers. She tried to understand the sufferings and brave journey of Divyansh by displaying her remarkable equanimity. When I told her that all his life, Divyansh had converted his pain into pleasure and used that to harness his own potential to counter the pain, she was quite moved and hugged Divyansh. Who knew that her new-found friend would become an inspiration to her at a later date! It is said that in a given time and space, whatever happens is destined; it happens for a purpose which may not be known when it happens. The meeting of Leuma and Divyansh was for a purpose. When we stood up to leave after we were done, she handed us a packed meal box to enjoy in our apartment. Gideon drove us back to our apartment and I, sitting by his side, was still trying to absorb all that we had experienced there. I looked at Divyansh in the side-mirror of the car. His eyes nodded at me conveying: Leuma is a paragon of virtue.

Back in the apartment after our visit, I found Divyansh in a thoughtful mood. He was trying to weave something in abstract. I reluctantly punctured his thoughts and asked, 'What's up?'

'The difficulties or challenges we get in our lives are not supposed to paralyse us. Rather they help us discover who we are and who all are accompanying us in helping to face the challenge. The struggle of mine is not only mine. A lot of persons including you, are rallying behind me and struggling in the same measure. Today, one more person is added to the list. And that's Leuma. I feel humbled by her,' Divyansh replied philosophically.

All night long, his golden words echoed in my ears. Divyansh was our parental responsibility. Leuma lent her helping hands in our pursuit.

Till we returned to Mumbai on 9 September 2015, we were in regular touch with Leuma. She always insisted we join her family on Sabbath Day and we never said no. Our bonding became stronger by the day. Her attachment to Divyansh also grew stronger because by that time, he had taken baby steps in speaking Hebrew language, which was fascinating to her. On the day we left, she sent her good wishes and expressed her desire to stay in touch.

We flew back to Mumbai on 9 September 2015 with fond memories of her.

Back home, Divyansh went into study mode for the upcoming Class 12 exams and, in between, visiting the local physician for follow-up treatment. We kept in contact with Leuma and her family through regular exchange of messages and occasional calls.

In the next year, Divyansh developed some post-transplantation complications due to which we had to travel to Jerusalem quite a few times. Meeting Leuma and her family was an added charm every time we visited Jerusalem. On our trip in August 2016, Leuma and Gideon came to visit us at our apartment, and took us to a café named Avichael, which was right below our apartment. She had brought a precious gift for Divyansh: a khamsa. A khamsa is a palm-shaped amulet popular across the Middle East, commonly used as wall-hangings. The Jews believe that it provides defence against evil eyes. Somewhere in her heart, Leuma was not happy with our repeated visits to Jerusalem. The visits were for the wrong reasons, she felt. She thought Divyansh needed some protection from evil eyes, and so she gifted him the khamsa. She was doing her best to shield Divyansh from evil forces. Divyansh was quite moved by the gift—more than the gift, the spirit behind her choosing it as a gift for him.

When we returned to Mumbai, Divyansh always kept this khamsa on his study table to soak himself uninterrupted in Leuma's motherly affection emanating from it.

We went back to Jerusalem supposedly for the last time on 18 September 2016. This time, Divyansh wanted to take a souvenir for Leuma. He went to the Colaba Market in Mumbai and he bought her an owl. He wished to add an owl sourced from India to her unique owl collection in the glass cabinet.

We were off to Jerusalem. As soon as the flight landed in Tel Aviv, a WhatsApp message dropped in my mobile. It read: 'Hi! Welcome to Jerusalem. Hope to meet you soon. Wish the treatment be effective and the result be health, health and health. I joined the club—an unexpected surprise...'

I couldn't understand what she meant by 'I joined the club'. On reaching our apartment, I called her to enquire about it. She said, 'I should have told you that humour is one of the weapons I use against the enemy. I have been diagnosed with cancer.'

I was stunned and remained mute for some time. After coming to terms with this awful shock, I shared the news with Divyansh.

He remained calm. And why not, life had taught him to deal with such situations with utmost poise. He didn't utter a word. After a while, he gave a blank smile which conveyed a lot, a lot more than his words would. A week later, Leuma and Gideon wanted to visit our apartment. We were quite happy to meet them. On the morning of 29 September, I saw Divyansh writing something on a piece of paper. I asked what he was writing. He said he was trying to pen some thoughts on Leuma. He wished to hand it over to her along with the souvenir when she would come to visit us in the evening.

Leuma and Gideon came over that evening. After sharing pleasantries, Divyansh gave Leuma first the owl, and then his handwritten letter. But before that, he read out the letter. Perhaps he wanted each and every word written by him to echo his emotions as he read. He wrote:

29 September 2016

Dear Mrs Leuma,

In India, when we want to address someone who is not our relative but older than us, we use the suffix of either 'Aunty' or 'Uncle' after their name to address them. So, I will address you as Leuma Aunty.

Dear Leuma Aunty,

All my family members, who have so far joined me in my medical and spiritual journey here in Israel, fail to recall many other local families we have been received by so hospitably. But no one forgets you, fondly recalling you as the sweet, ebullient, mother-like 'aunty' who loves owls.

It was only later in my stay here in Israel, that I had the fortune of meeting godly souls like you and Gideon Uncle. I feel so loved, secure and blessed to have the pleasure of knowing angels like you.

The care and support, both physical and more importantly mental, you have given us will forever make us indebted to you and will always receive blessings from us whenever you appear in our consciousness.

What has happened with you is most unfortunate. And I, personally, know the deep sorrow and fear of the unknown you must be going through despite putting up such a brave and calm face. It is perfectly normal. I just wish I could do for you what you have done for me, so far. But my capabilities are limited. What I can offer you humbly is advice and promise to be your cheer brigade whenever you feel sad, upset, not well or just not right.

First of all, I will advise you to *accept* your current situation as soon as you can. This is like a bitter pill, the longer you take to swallow it, the more unpleasant it will feel. 'Yes, I have this problem. The problem is in my body. The problem is not in me. I have a disease. I am not diseased,' should be your mantra.

Next, you take a spoonful of *denial*—sweet denial. But do this after the first step. This sweet syrup will take out all the bitterness and help you go about living your yofe (very nice) life as if nothing has happened at all. Go to the gym like you do, wear that sporty swimwear and swim like a mermaid, go and meet your friends regularly, help others like you have always been doing and, most importantly, don't change even ounce of yourself. Continue being the lovely adorable angel you are.

There will be tough days—if not many, some for sure. But I am sure a strong and tough person like you will triumph over them. Just one advice—*don't let these bad days go to your head*. Ignore poisonous thoughts stemming on these days. Talk to friends. Chat with closed ones. I am also there!

Since you are strong and an implicit believer in God,

pray to Him whenever you can, and remember Him whenever you feel weak. But also trust your own mental strength and believe strongly in yourself.

> Sweet are the uses of adversity.
> Which like the toad, ugly and venomous
> Wears yet a precious jewel in his head.

An apt quote on adversity by William Shakespeare. It took me several years of grooming up to grasp its true essence. I firmly believe in this and am giving this quote to you. I would like to say Mazel Tov. Your misfortune is going to make you stronger! You will undergo a new rediscovery and learn new things about yourself. You will imbibe new qualities in yourself, all good ones. Trust me; this has been my experience so far.

Attached with this well-meant letter is a small token of my gratitude for you. Please open it.

The owl, in our religion, is the vehicle of Goddess Lakshmi, the goddess of wealth and prosperity. It is also the vehicle of the Greek goddess Athena, the goddess of wisdom. May you be blessed by both these goddesses. You will always remain in my prayers.

Lechaim and Betzlakha!

Yours truly,

Divyansh

As Divyansh read out his letter, I saw Leuma, in complete awe, listening intently and trying to absorb each and every word spoken by him.

Leuma must have read that letter a few times more before texting a message to Divyansh the next day:

My Dear Divyansh,

I read and re-read what you wrote and I find it wonderful. You are wise, brave and noble-minded. You share your insight so clearly and convincing I am thankful for that. In addition, I am sure and pray and wish that you are going to win your battle and come out healthy and strong and that success is waiting for you in whatever you choose to do. I feel very happy and lucky to know you and your family. Thanks and I love you.

Leuma

We returned to Mumbai towards the end of October. We had to go to Jerusalem one last time towards the end of December that year for a couple of days. We met Leuma and it appeared that she was not responding to the treatment. But she wore a spirited look.

Back in Mumbai, Divyansh had resumed his classes at his engineering college. Leuma and Divyansh were always in touch.

Fortune was not by Divyansh's side. His condition began to deteriorate towards the beginning of March 2017. We purposely didn't share the news with Leuma as she herself was in a poor condition. We feared sharing the news would dampen her spirit to fight for her own life. While Divyansh was undergoing treatment in USA, I got a message from her daughter, Orna conveying the sad news of Leuma passing away in the first week of June. On hearing this, Divyansh just closed his eyes and it seemed he was trying to experience the mighty Leuma in his soul and conveying his condolences. Divyansh still carried her khamsa, through which he always imagined Leuma protecting him from evil eyes.

Divyansh had torrid days ahead and underwent painful suffering since October 2017, before finally bidding us good bye on 2 May 2019.

The khamsa, this time too, tried to protect him from his deep

sufferings and transported him to a better world, a world where
he could meet his soulmate, Leuma.

Savdas

We reached Jerusalem on 30 March 2015. After checking into the
apartment, we straightway proceeded to the Hadassah Hospital
where Divyansh was to undergo treatment. Rajesh Parihar, an
IFS officer who worked at the Indian Consulate office in Tel Aviv
and who knew our travel plan, came to visit us on the very first
day—first hour—at the hospital. My acquaintance with Rajesh was
hardly a few days old, and we had come into contact through
a common friend. I felt humbled by his gesture of coming over
to the hospital, driving about 70 km, all the way from Tel Aviv.
He was with us all day long and attempted to understand our
immediate needs. He informed me about a gentleman named
Savdas, who also lived in Tel Aviv, who could be of great help
to us. He immediately connected me to Savdas over the phone.

Savdas was a person of Indian origin who had been in Israel
since 1993 and was now an Israeli citizen. He lived in Peteh
Tikva near Jerusalem. He had a beautiful family consisting of
his wife, Reena, and three children. He ran an Indian grocery
store in Tel Aviv, and also installed security systems in business
establishments on the side. He spoke Hebrew so fluently that
it was very difficult to differentiate him from the native people
speaking the language. He seemed to have seamlessly blended in
the socio-cultural mainstream of the country.

When we had planned to visit Jerusalem, we carried minimum
Indian groceries, fearing immigration problems in Israel. Eating
daily from a restaurant was out of question because, first,
Divyansh had to be fed with home-cooked food and, second,
the foods served in their restaurants were completely different
from our staple diet. Therefore, what we instantly needed there

was eclectic varieties of Indian groceries. Savdas readily offered his benevolence. It is important to understand that the typical Indian groceries were very difficult to find in stores there. However, later during our stay, we discovered some shops selling a few Indian spices and pulses.

Savdas took our provision requirements through text message. The very next day he visited us, driving 70 km from Tel Aviv with two big bags, one containing groceries as requested by me and the other containing plenty of home-cooked food, sent by his compassionate wife. I was bowled over by him that day. I politely told him, 'I am feeling hugely embarrassed to accept food sent by your wife. I appreciate her sense of kindness to us. Since you have brought it today, I must accept this with all humility, but please, from next time, avoid.' He listened to me nonchalantly and then he started talking about Mumbai. I offered him money for the groceries he had brought, which he politely refused. Despite pestering him hard, he refused to take money and told me to text him whenever we needed more in future. Those were my early days in managing affairs of the kitchen. Nevertheless, I offered him a cup of tea, to which he said that he didn't drink tea.

The cooked food sent by my wife, Nidhi, had been almost completely consumed by us by then. Before Savdas came, I was struggling with what to cook. It appeared, then, a Herculean task for me to cook food, as all my life, I had never cooked. And one can always blame me for that. I regretted it then. And then, Savdas came with a bag full of home-cooked food, the kind of food we would have been served had Nidhi been with us. We relished that food for the next three days, and by then, I started taking baby steps in cooking. I still cherish the magnanimity of Savdas and the thoughtfulness of his wife when I reminisce about that day.

One remarkable feature I found in Savdas was that he never said no to any request made or help asked of him. And to top that, he always appeared unassuming after each such act of benevolence from him. Throughout our stay there, I had to source Indian groceries from him several times and he always obliged us instantly. His hunger to serve us always outweighed our need of those things. I knew that he would not accept money for his supplies every time and I was infected with guilt, but he, over a period of time, became so dependable and close to our hearts that sourcing these goods from elsewhere felt like a colossal sin to me. The relationship that we shared did not allow me to explore other people for the same services or the market to source them despite recurrent guilt.

Many a time, Savdas invited us for dinner to his home where his wife served us a lavish spread of Indian cuisine. Invariably, after dinner, Savdas would drive us back to our apartment. He made it a point to visit us even when there was no requirement of any supplies.

In our subsequent visit to Jerusalem, I once enquired about a place called Elat, which was a four-hour drive from our apartment. Elat was a southern Israeli port and resort town on the Red Sea. Its beaches were noted for their calm waters. It was also known for snorkelling and diving. Coral Beach Natural Reserve had underwater trails among fish-filled reefs. It was famous for the Coral World Underwater Observatory. I wanted to show Divyansh this place. By then, Divyansh had visited all the important places in Israel except Elat. How could Savdas have shied away from this responsibility? He gracefully extended his courtesy, driving us to Elat, staying with us there and finally dropping us back at our apartment.

As long as we were in Jerusalem, his goodness kept coming to us, shining through his benevolent acts. It was quite moving for us. Savdas is still in touch with us and still tries to extend his helping hands, even though Divyansh now rests in eternal tranquillity.

Dear Savdas, you are a true epitome of the global religion—humanity—as envisioned by Divyansh.

David

Dear Sushil,

Shalom.

When you answered and not Div, I thought something was up. I am very sorry. Div tried to speak to me when he was at Hadassah to get his immunotherapy. It was after I left the hospital and I was in severe depression, if you can believe it. I think I shunned Div at that time and I feel bad about it. I am okay now, off medication for one-and-a-half years. Is he responsive? Did you play my birthday card message to him? I wish I could be there with you. Give him a big hug for me. All the best to my buddy, Div.

David   28 January 2019

We knew David J. Dembrow even before we started our journey to Jerusalem. He was a well-known nurse at the Hadassah Hospital, who had earlier attended to Divyansh's school friend during his treatment. A year of service was left before his retirement when we came in contact with him. I clearly remember the day when Divyansh and I had met him in the BMT department after consultation with Dr Reuven Or. Clad in white nurses' dress, with a saline bottle in his hand, he smiled profusely when we introduced ourselves and referred to Divyansh's friend. David instantly remembered him and, pointing to a room, said that he was treated in that room. He felt as if that room was lucky and, therefore, he would ensure Divyansh got that room whenever he was admitted. His sublime smile evoked affection for us to soak in. There was not much of interaction on that day as he was on duty.

On the day Divyansh was admitted to the ward where David worked, he prayed to get David as his room nurse. There were 20 rooms in that ward and each nurse was assigned three–four rooms to attend to the patients. David was not on duty in that shift and, so, Divyansh was attended by a lady nurse, Netah, who appeared quite proficient in her work. Soon, the day came when David was assigned Divyansh's room to attend to. And then, the saga of their relationship ensued. Gradually, both of them started bonding. I later found Divyansh's areas of interest matched almost perfectly with those of David. They talked about on going soccer matches, tennis Grand Slams, upcoming US presidential elections, food, culture and what not. Divyansh played his playlist on the bluetooth speaker which enthralled David. The chief nurse of the ward, Yevgeni, was a smart person with a humane face. He immediately sensed the growing relationship between Divyansh and David and, also, perhaps David's preference to be assigned his room, though, as a professional, he couldn't choose a particular patient to serve. But Yevgeni always ensured he assigned Divyansh's room to David in his shift. Their affinity for each other and association gained strength day by day. The treatment process was tough, painful and, perhaps, life-threatening. Divyansh confessed to me later that but for David, it wouldn't have been a smooth sail. Quite often, I found David sitting with Divyansh after attending to all his patients, engaged in spirited conversation with him, rather than sitting at the nurse station. Divyansh now became Div for David.

I, as a father, marvelled at the intensity of their friendship and their understanding and appreciation for each other's thoughts. It occurred to me that there was some divinity attached to their relationship. Divyansh, while fighting against his nemesis, couldn't stay in touch with his friends. They were there, but not when they really mattered to him. He was alone. Over a period of time, I tried to befriend him beyond the realm of a father–son relationship. I must have shared a lot of my personal matters, hitherto not known to him, just to make him comfortable and ease him enough to open his cards in the same way. Divyansh did reciprocate my initiative. But at the end of the day, our attempted friendship could never come out of the domain of the father–son dynamic. His growing friendship with David gave succour to me. What was remarkable to note was that their age difference of almost of 50 years wasn't any impediment in establishing sterling chemistry between them. It is said that a real friend is one who walks in when the rest of the world walks out. With David, Divyansh was redefining the contours of bonhomie around a friend. Thus, he found new arsenal in the form of David in his quiver, with which he was able to tread on his path with remarkable poise.

After the conclusion of the treatment, we planned to return on 9 September 2015. Divyansh had something in his mind before we embarked on our journey back to Mumbai. Two days before the journey, Divyansh wished to meet David in the hospital. Respecting his sentiment, I took him to the hospital. David was too busy on duty that day. Somehow, he squeezed in some time to meet Divyansh outside the ward. After exchanging a few pleasantries, Divyansh gracefully gave an envelope to David requesting him to read his note in leisure. I, a mute spectator there, watched their adoring eye contact with a straight face.

Divyansh wrote:

A friend in need is a friend indeed.

I have only recently understood the true meaning of this quote. And now that I have understood its essence, I found it quite fitting to use it for the friend who revealed to me its true meaning.

I am writing this letter especially for you, David, because of all the nurses, I found you to be the most special one. This I am confiding to you in private, because I want to keep it that way—implicit and tacit. You may be almost the age of my grandparents, but such is your personality that I always felt as if I was talking to one of my 'bros', one of my 'mates'. The most wonderful thing about you is the energy you exude that instantly recharges anyone in your vicinity, no matter how down they may be. Your efficiency, dedication and attention to the tiniest of details are truly uniquely special, or rather, classy. Of course, there is also your sense of humour. But there is one thing I experienced only in your presence, not discrediting or taking away any other nurse's credit—I could not help but smile with happiness in your presence and jump with joy internally every morning I saw you walking through those doors with my 'morning goodies', saying, 'Hey bud! How are you?'

Dear David, I will cherish every moment that you nursed me, every moment when you made me laugh, every moment of joy I felt with you as my nurse in my most difficult times, the pains you took to tie and untie the plastic around the PICC line, the pains you took to shove three–four IV bags in and out of the sleeve so that I am 100 per cent safe and every lesson of life that I learnt from you. You are my new best friend and a true 'cool dude'. Goodbye.

Your 'bud',
Divyansh Atman

David replied on the same day on Divyansh's Facebook wall. He wrote:

Divyansh,

Shalom. Just wanted you to know that I read your letter on the way home. It brought tears to my eyes. I [have been] in the BMT department for many years, as you know. It is, without a doubt, the most precious gift I have ever received. I feel we have truly bonded. It will truly be a keepsake for many years.

Divyansh came back to Mumbai on 9 September with the sweet memory of his new best friend and true 'cool dude', David. He got busy in Mumbai making up for his lost studies for the upcoming board examination. He remained in touch with David through messages and occasional calls. One day, Divyansh's friend, whom David had also treated, came home to meet him. Divyansh clicked a photograph together with his friend and sent it to David with a comment, 'Got this picture clicked especially for you. Please show it to all your colleagues.' David replied, 'I don't believe my eyes. Too much to say. This picture, I will cherish, all my days.' When I read his reply, it was an immensely humbling experience. Divyansh wrote, 'When you look at this photo, feel good because you have contributed to bringing this smile on our faces.'

David was due to retire in January 2016. The BMT department was planning to organize a send-off party for him. The chief nurse of the BMT department, Yevgeni, wanted to give David a priceless gift. He had his own plan. He texted Divyansh in early January to record his thoughts on David in a video clip which he wanted to play on a giant screen at the farewell party. The idea was good and exhilarating. When David must have treated tens of thousands of patients in his career spanning almost 40 years, I wondered why Yevgeni chose Divayansh amongst all. Maybe he knew Divyansh had become Div for David. Together, they had given a new meaning to the patient–nurse relationship. Yevgeni was sentimentally mindful of their relationship. Even otherwise, for a nurse, the most befitting persons to give a farewell speech are the patients whom he/she serves.

This offer Divyansh grabbed with both hands. He prepared his speech and I video-recorded as he spoke, clad in a bright yellow T-shirt. The video clip was sent to Yevgeni. After the send-off party, Yevgeni sent us the video footage of the function. I was in complete amazement to see everyone present there in tears as Divyansh appeared on the giant screen, giving his speech for

David. They were stunned. David was astounded. It appeared he didn't believe his eyes at what he was witnessing. And why not? That was straight from Div to David. In his long speech, Divyansh made one remarkable comment which really summed up David as a person and a nurse: 'For people who come to your ward for treatment, you are a beautiful gift. You make their tough journey a joyful and easy one.'

While giving this speech, which I recorded, I felt Divyansh wanted to say a lot more. He had to stop. What he couldn't say was that David would always remain conspicuous by his absence in the BMT department of the Hadassah Hospital hereafter.

Call to go back to Jerusalem again.

Divyansh developed some complications post treatment. We planned our visit to Jerusalem in April 2016 for a check-up. He was elated to make the most of the trip by also meeting David.

After reaching Jerusalem, Divyansh texted David to meet. It seemed David was preoccupied. He expressed his inability to come. There were few more message exchanges between them to materialize the meeting but in vain. David could not make it. Divyansh was craving to meet him. He kept trying to meet him in subsequent visits to Jerusalem too, but didn't succeed. There was complete silence from David's side. Sometimes, silence speaks louder than words. Perhaps Divyansh was hearing those unspoken words. People close to Divyansh know that his personality was like sand on a beach. It would withstand all sorts of waves—gentle or tormenting—and remain grounded after each gush of waves, soaking in all the water.

Divyansh stopped bothering David anymore. He moved on with his life, from Jerusalem to Mumbai and then to USA, where he fulfilled his dream of studying in a prestigious university there. Unfortunately, the disease relapsed for the last time with irreversible complications. He was brought back to India to spend his last few days at his home. Divyansh was hardly interacting.

On his twenty-second birthday on 27 January 2019, there was a voice message in Divyansh's mobile. I checked it. Life springs a lot of surprises. It gives enough opportunities to redeem what one has lost.

That voice message was David greeting Divyansh on his birthday. He didn't know what had happened to him till then. However, the way David spoke, it seemed like he was trying to wake Divyansh from his trance. I played the voice message to him. He did try to connect with that. How far, only the two friends knew. I couldn't stop my tears. David had to be told the truth. I texted him and narrated the whole story. He replied that when I had answered to his voice message instead of Divyansh, he immediately thought there was something seriously wrong with him. He expressed his regret for his inability to respond to Divyansh's call when he had come to Jerusalem for his immunotherapy, as he was suffering from severe depression then. Remorsefully, he asked me to give him a big hug and wish him happy birthday and good luck for his health.

Divyansh moved on to another world. But before that, David touched him again. It was a moment of redemption for David and his friendship with Divyansh. Maybe it was Divyansh's wish before he could say goodbye to him. David fulfilled that.

On Divyansh's first birthday in his new world on 27 Januray 2020, of all his friends, only one greeted him on his Facebook wall. That was David. He wrote: 'Div hey! It's your day. Time to celebrate, which I am sure you are doing. Have a very Heavenly Birthday. Can't wait to see you, Bro.'

Dear David and Div, *Mazel tov l'chaim*! Long live your friendship.

Navdeep Singh

August 2018. A person came all the way from Kosovo to see Divyansh in a hospital in Mumbai. The cure for his condition was beyond the realm of medical science, as repeatedly recited to us by the doctors. Recited, because we were tired of hearing the same narrative for the past ten months: first in USA and now in Mumbai. We had not yet given up. As soon as Divyansh saw that person, he cried. Actually he did cry, more with his eyes than with his face. He wanted to say something to him but couldn't. The person just could not take it anymore. He lovingly caressed Divyansh's cheek with his right hand and left the room with tears in his eyes. We were awestruck.

Navdeep Singh, a gentleman to the core from Delhi, was a part of the Indian diaspora who had been working in the United Nation Truce Supervision Office (UNTSO) in Jerusalem as an engineer since 2005. He lived there with his family consisting of his home-maker wife and three children, the youngest being a cute, adorable son. We didn't know each other before I went to Jerusalem. I heard about him through a common friend. His nobility can be gauged from the fact that as soon as he learnt of our plan to visit Jerusalem for Divyansh's treatment, he called me and tried to understand our requirements for our stay and logistics. We had never been to Israel in the past. He swiftly arranged a decent, comfortable and economical apartment nearby, paid the advance and booked a slot for us. Divyansh, in his six years of battle with his nemesis, had evolved a lot. Every couple of years, the direction of his life changed as a result of relapse and connected medical problems and his old mates would leave his company as his path changed. Divyansh, on a new path, would evolve more, tread alone, radiating fresh wisdom and positivity and then would form a new caravan as he progressed. Who knew then that Navdeep, one of the most recent additions in his caravan, would not leave him, no matter how many times his life changed its path, in this life or beyond.

When we reached Jerusalem, Navdeep was in Europe on a family trip. By the time we settled down in the city with the help of new-found friends like Soshi, Michelle and Caron, the outline on the process became clearer and we could figure out the broad contours of our stay there. Navdeep met us at our apartment the day he returned from the tour. I can't forget that day: he was in a black jacket as the day was cold then. He sat with us and talked in great detail about our family and our immediate necessities in Jerusalem. It was our first meeting. His very presence was comforting with his well-poised demeanour. Before leaving, he said he would soon invite us to dinner at his home. The very first meeting with him gave us a feeling that he was going to be a selfless champion of our support system there. Many a time he drove to our apartment and took us to dinner at his home, where his wife, Deepa, served us traditional Indian foods prepared with great alacrity. We used to sit in his house for hours, as we had time since the treatment process hadn't begun yet. After the dinner, he would religiously drive us back to our apartment. Our bond was becoming more and more informal now, and we could talk on any subject without inhibition. I could see Divyansh slowly develop a liking for him and his family, and would quite often engage in soulful conversation with him. Divyansh was still in his teens, precisely 18 years old, but diffused the aura of a mature person, much beyond his age. Navdeep was apparently charmed by his persona.

One day, Navdeep, in his unassuming words, told me something which was the most humbling experience in my life. Our relationship was still in the budding stages which had just begun on a time scale. But he found it blossoming, and that's why he told me unhesitatingly about his wish to extend his monetary support to me in our trying times. He felt that this was the least he could do for me, which I shouldn't refuse. Although I politely refused the offer with heartfelt thanks, I could not deny his profound spirit behind this support, more valuable than his money, which has found permanent abode in my heart.

Divyansh had been a keen student in his school days and later in his life as well. One day, Navdeep called us to show us the UN office. It was like a dream come true for Divyansh. Not just Divyansh, it was exciting and enticing for me too. Navdeep showed us every nook and corner of the campus. Whatever we had studied about the UN in Social Sciences was being played out right before us. It was a strange feeling, difficult to describe in words. Later, Divyansh told me that he got a sublime feeling, seeing pan world-view when he visited the Central Hall, where flags of member countries were hoisted. He felt very proud to have seen the Indian flag amongst the rest. Whilst leaving the campus, Navdeep showed us a small retreat, made for the officers where they spent time during 'happy hours' on Friday. This place later carried a significant importance in the annals of my relationship with Divyansh.

When the treatment process was due to commence, Nidhi and my daughter Ananya also joined us. That was the time Deepa became her unconditional support system. She regularly interacted with Nidhi to let her unwind from the rigours of medical treatment. She often sent cooked food for us during our hospital days. Honestly, we were embarrassed to see them taking such pains for us. Navdeep and his family had become a solid support pillar we could always lean against. As long as Nidhi and Ananya were there, Navdeep ensured that they were always kept engaged in one way or another.

The sixty-eighth Independence Day of our country was round the corner. Nidhi and Ananya had left for Mumbai. Divyansh didn't want to miss the celebration of this big day. He asked me if it was possible to visit the Indian Consulate at Tel Aviv to witness the Independence Day celebration. The idea was good. I knew a few people in the consulate office. Divyansh was recuperating after the treatment. His low immunity was an issue in my decision whether to take him to Tel Aviv or not. I broached the subject with Navdeep to solicit his advice. He came up with another plan. The next morning, he himself came to pick us up from the apartment and drove us to the Indian Consulate at Tel Aviv. Attending Independence Day celebration away from the country amongst the Indian diaspora was a unique feeling, never experienced before. When the national anthem was being sung in chorus on foreign soil, with each '*jaya he, jaya he*', we felt goosebumps erupt all over our arms. Divyansh considered himself fortuitous having made it to this occasion. I silently thanked Navdeep for helping me discharge my fatherly responsibility. After the celebration was over, Navdeep took us to an exquisite tourist spot, Ros Haniqra, about 130 km away from Tel Aviv. While returning, he took even more pains to take us to Haifa, a port city. He drove all day long before finally dropping us to our apartment. I, as a husband and a father, was always conscious of the feelings of his wife and children who may have wanted to spend this day with him. It is said that when you come to a point where you have no need to impress anybody, your freedom will begin. Navdeep's spirit had attained that freedom. It was his unconditional care for us.

Time was ticking away. It was time to return to Mumbai after the treatment. Divyansh was very happy. For so many days, he had missed his mummy and darling sister Ananya. It was a moment of exhilaration for Navdeep too. Navdeep was known for expressing measured emotions. That's how he was. But those few measured emotional words were enough to indicate how happy he was on the successful completion of Divyansh's treatment and our impending family reunion.

Off to Mumbai.

Early March next year, some unfamiliar symptoms started

bothering Divyansh. With those symptoms, he somehow appeared for the Class 12 board examination and, to our amazement, was ranked amongst the top five in his college. After finishing the exams, we again visited to Jerusalem for a follow-up. As before, Navdeep made our stay arrangements, but in a different place. Food was an issue there, but Navdeep made sure that Divyansh always got custom-made food from his kitchen. This, despite the fact that he had to attend to office work from 7 a.m. to 3 p.m., Monday to Friday. He took good care of Divyansh not only outside the hospital but also in the hospital, by always being with us. We felt completely devastated to see Divyansh struggle with new complications. Navdeep was with me all the time to fall back on. The doctor advised Divyansh to undergo one specialized infusion of medicine after a month. We prepared to come back. Navadeep came to the hotel to meet us. Before leaving, Divyansh handed an envelope to him requesting him to open it after our departure. I didn't have any occasion to know what it contained. On the way, Divyansh told me that he had written a letter to Navdeep to express his gratitude. Four years down the line, when I sat down to pen our golden memories with Navdeep, I wanted to read that letter to reflect. I texted Navdeep to ask if he still had that letter, and if he did, could he send me a copy of that? Navdeep sent me images of the three-page letter and the envelope on WhatsApp with the following message, 'Sending the letter with tears. Makes me feel helpless and don't know what I could have done better to have him with us...'

The letter and the envelope looked as fresh as they did in April 2016 when it was given to Navdeep. He had treasured this letter with great care. That's why he could send it immediately. I read Divyansh's golden words now, which I hadn't when these were written. I couldn't stop my tears. He had written two letters, one addressed to Navdeep and the other, very thoughtfully, to his wife Deepa.

Here is an excerpt from the letter addressed to Navdeep:

In school, we first read about the UN. We read and study about the different roles of the organization, the different specialized sub-organs and how it almost works as the caretaker of the world, rising above the physical and mental borders we have divided our world into. You, Uncle, are true embodiment of the above—coming out of nowhere and going miles and poles apart to convert our relationship into something strong and beautiful.

An excerpt from the letter addressed to Deepa:

There are people who pretend to help you. There are people who only want to show how much concern they have for you. I have seen countless such people through my trying times. But you and Uncle are the rare genuine angels, the warm, yet rock solid support, who transcend the borders of family to provide unknown people like us your lovely home. This, for me, makes you beacon lights of nobility far and wide.

To me, these were golden words of gratitude expressed by Divyansh. Perhaps I should have also done this then. Divyansh's life span was not long but it was big. He unknowingly did so many things that demonstrated his keenness to shoulder his father's responsibilities. Maybe this letter was one of those acts, I realize in hindsight.

There is a big difference between sympathy and empathy at a psychological level. Navdeep always empathized with us without showing any sign of sympathy. That's the hallmark of a good human being.

On our next visit to Jerusalem in early July 2016 for the specialized treatment, Navdeep picked up from where he had left off. He again expressed his desire to extend some financial help to me. I politely said no and became more obliged in the face of his nobility. That was the time I had gone there with my sister-in-law, Shikha, who was very close to Divyansh. The treatment started as per the plan, which was to be taken uninterruptedly for one month. One Friday, Navdeep proposed to take us to his UN office to enjoy happy hours on the campus. Divyansh was frank enough to join us in the happy hours. That was the day I had a drink with Navdeep, perhaps for the first time in Jerusalem. But more importantly, it was the first time I had a drink in the presence of Divyansh. He knew that I drank occasionally and was quite comfortable with it. But I never did it in his presence. That day, with glass of whisky in my hand, I cheered with him. The whisky drew us closer. The happy hours took our father–son relationship to a higher pedestal, more informal than it had been.

One day, while Divyansh's treatment was still going on, my eldest brother called me from my native place, Patna, informing me about my father's (Babooji) serious illness. He was later shifted to the ICU after his medical condition worsened. And then, he was finally put on life support system. His life, then, had taken refuge in the machine. Divyansh's life had taken refuge in me there in Jerusalem. I was at crossroads, with a gigantic moral crisis. If I flew to Patna to see my Babooji, I would have to leave Divyansh alone. And if I didn't, I would have a life-long regret of not seeing him when it mattered the most. Babooji had immense faith in my prowess to manage his medical crisis. I had done so quite a few times for him in the past. I thought that he, on life support, must have been waiting for me to come and to give one more shot to ensure a fresh lease of his life. It pained me enormously to not have made it. Divyansh was well aware of my mental disharmony caused by the inner conflict. He, time and again, advised me to go to Patna with an assurance that he would manage in my absence. Amidst this inner conflict, I got the news of Babooji's death one morning a few days later. It was too much for me to control my emotional outburst. The tears were not only for Babooji's death but also for not managing to see him in his last hours.

Divyansh finally exercised his last writ. He held me tightly and almost ordered me to fly to Patna to attend the last rites. But how could I leave him alone? There came Navdeep again. He not only managed my return air tickets, but quietly told me to leave the responsibility of looking after Divyansh to him. On his assurance, I left Divyansh to the care of Navdeep and Shikha, and flew to Patna to attend the last rites. Navdeep, along with Shikha, handled his medical management in my absence. In retrospect, I realize now that I would not have been able to attend the last rites of Babooji had Navdeep not come to my rescue and had Divyansh not exercised his writ.

We visited Jerusalem again in October for the same treatment. Navdeep, as usual, was always with us. By that time Navdeep had decided to leave Jerusalem and join the UN office in Pristina, Kosovo, at a higher rank. When we came to Jerusalem for the last time in December, he was all set to shift his family to Kosovo. He had timed his departure with the end of our stay in Jerusalem.

We came back from our last visit of Jerusalem during Christmas in 2016. Early that year, Divyansh had joined an engineering college in Mumbai to pursue his dream to study Computer Science. He resumed the college and was in full steam there. He had once participated in a MUN in his college, in which he had represented Israel and made his noteworthy deliberations. He, after returning from the college, had shared the MUN badge with Navdeep with great joy. In the evening, he had a long insightful discussion with Navdeep regarding various roles of the UN vis-à-vis Israel.

Divyansh was in full swing in his college, making friends and enjoying college life. And then, the final blow. He relapsed for the last time and the only treatment which was available was in trial stage in USA. We flew to USA for his treatment. It is said that the best success habit is being trained to handle failures. Divyansh knew how to achieve success amidst hardship. He always utilized moments of hardship as an opportunity to explore himself. Such pains always drove him to the path of redemption. While taking treatment in USA, he ensured his admission in a university in New Jersey in Electrical Engineering with full scholarship. When Navdeep heard about it, he was very happy and sent a congratulatory message to Divyansh. Divyansh seemed to manage his studies and medical issues alongside. But over the next four months, he developed some irreversible complications. He had to be hospitalized there for a long time. Navdeep constantly remained in touch and kept offering what he could at that stage apart from empathizing: the monetary help, which I again declined. Finally, considering his deteriorating medical condition, we brought Divyansh to Mumbai to spend his last few months at home, with his own. But before bringing him to home, we first admitted him to a hospital in Mumbai for two weeks of rehabilitation.

Navdeep called me from Kosovo and informed me that he was coming to Mumbai to see Divyansh. I couldn't stop him. By then, Divyansh belonged as much to him as to me. In August 2018, he visited Divyansh in the hospital. It appeared that Divyansh wanted to say something to Navdeep but couldn't. Navdeep couldn't hold himself and went out of the room to regain his composure.

Months later, Divyansh moved to a new world on 2 May 2019. Navdeep shared his thoughts on Divyansh with me:

> Words can't fulfil the vacuum being created with his absence despite [the fact that] I was physically away from him. Hope and miracle were the two words I always had in my prayers for Divyansh. His pain was felt each day despite our long distance. One day, we all will leave this world but his departure left a big void in the lives of all his near and dear ones. Divyansh as a son, brother, friend, noble soul

will always remain in memories until we all will meet him again in our next journey. Despite the unbearable pain he was going through when I met him last August, he wanted to ask, 'Uncle, how are you?'

You have left us all with memories and the pain forever...
I love you and miss you until we will meet one day...

Navdeep is still in touch with me and also with Divyansh in his new life.

EPILOGUE

With time, I have realized every bit of Divyansh in me in whatever I do now. Though I am still grieving, he has made me realize my own existential meaning. I began reading a lot of books, especially those recommended by him. As long as I read books, I feel Divyansh is with me. During this process I was driven to my own actualization. Gradually, a thought began driving me into weaving a story based on his inspirational life journey. In the process of drafting this book, I could unravel his virtues, actions and mental fortitude in a new way. I came back to many aspects of his personality and actions, which I thought I had understood, and while creating this book, I saw much deeper meaning in them. My own life's journey with him has made me see my life in a different way. I must be one of those rare parents who is writing a biographical story of her own son and who has idolized him so much that she is inspirationally following his footsteps. This book is an attempt by me along with Sushil to give a new birth to my son and make him immortal. Like him, it had been a catharsis for me all through the journey of making of this book.

Two months after Divyansh's passing away, we learnt that his alma mater St. Mary's School (ICSE), Mumbai, instituted a scholarship named 'Divyansh Atman Scholarship for Creative Writing' in his memory. We were invited to give away the scholarship and certificates to the well-deserving students at their award function on 20 July 2019. Before announcing the institution of the scholarship, a PowerPoint presentation was made on the inspiring journey and creative excellence of Divyansh. After that, we were called up to the dais to give away the certificates of excellence to the recipients. As we walked slowly to the dais, the packed auditorium gave us a standing ovation. I couldn't hold my tears. Those claps were not for me; they were for Divyansh. During the break, the vice-principal of the school told us she still felt Divyansh's presence in the school even after so many years.

Divyansh had been a regular participant in the Mumbai chapter of a global movement, 100TPC. In the past, his poem 'Blaze' was published in its annual compilation. The Mumbai chapter dedicated the poetry festival of 2019 to Divyansh, where Sushil and I were invited to release a book titled *The Miracle of Life*, in which 'Blaze' was published again along with a brief account of his life journey. As we went up to the dais to inaugurate the book, I found my son everywhere amidst the roaring claps from the audience.

The poems that Divyansh wrote were read by several people, both in India and abroad, some of whom, out of their appreciation for it, took copies of 'Here We Go Again' in USA. His literary work needed to be protected from possible plagiarism. We got all of Divyansh's literary work copyrighted in November 2019. When we got the copyright certificate, we found our names printed as the owners of his literary work. It seems our names are permanently etched in all his literary work.

Ananya passed her Class 10 board exams with good marks. As I write this book, she is a student at Sophia College, Mumbai, in her second year. I must appreciate her as she has been able to bear with the pain of losing her brother in a remarkable way.

Sushil began writing about Divyansh and his association with several people whose lives he had touched in a big way, more importantly, those in Israel. I had to include as an integral part of this book the reminiscence that he wrote on Dr Reuven Or, the nurse David, Leuma, Navdeep Singh and Savdas because it is testimony to this fact. All these people are still in touch with us. In fact, Jenny and Zafi visited our home in January 2020 to reflect on the time they had spent with Divyansh. Dr Reuven Or keeps calling us regularly, and his contribution in making this book a reality can't be forgotten.

Just 10 days after Divyansh had passed away, Abhinav came to greet me on the Mother's Day on 12 May 2019 with a bouquet and gifted me a blank canvas to express my emotions on it. All the other therapists, namely, Zainab, Pallavi, Mansi, Fatema and Ms Roshan Vania, are regularly in touch and we interact with each other on a WhatsApp group called 'Divyansh Reverberation'. I now wear the kada Abhinav had given to Divyansh to wear.

Delzad came to visit us many times before going to USA for higher studies. He made sure to meet us just before his travel to New York. I gifted him a cap and a watch of Divyansh's. He communicates with us regularly and feels concerned for our well-being.

Ms Rati Wadia now teaches my daughter and makes every attempt to heal me spiritually. In the 2020 edition of the 100TPC, she read out Divyansh's poem 'The Tree of Purity'.

I can never forget Divyansh's twenty-third birthday, which fell on 27 January 2020. All his therapists came to meet us that evening and stayed with us till late at night. I realized they had come to celebrate his life.

The journey that Divyansh had started in Israel is yet to be completed. His seed is still stored in the sperm bank of the hospital there. Again, I am reminded of a thought—one doesn't go to Israel, he returns there.

AND HE LIVES ON

Catharsis

Hey God!
The Creator, the Sustainer, the Destroyer,
Today, I stand before You,
With reverence for your Supremacy,
And complete cluelessness about your next move.

Of course, I am too small a mortal,
To try to understand your Grand Design,
So I will say this to you straight,
And then bow my head, in grace.

I know you have your own plans for me,
I know, too, the whimsical, topsy-turvy nature of fate and destiny,
So I have decided now, to follow the words you had given humanity,
Sitting in that chariot, in the battlefield.

"Karmany evadhikaras te,
Ma phalesu kadachana,
Ma karma-phala-hetur bhur,
Ma te sango 'stv-akarmani"

I will do my karma,
I will carve my destiny,
I will now take control of my life, taking everything as it comes,
While relinquishing the dependence on fate,
And that Lady who calls herself Luck.

You are the Supreme Being,
Whom I will worship every day,
But neither will I ask You for anything,
Nor come to You with expectations.
I will sing Your praises,
I will find You in my soul,
But I will neither question You,
Nor the ways of Your works.

I will have unconditional implicit faith,
In your Grand design,
And never blame You, or fate,
For misfortune that may become mine.

I will wield my own plough,
I will cultivate my own land,
I will do all my karma,
And embrace whatever comes, with warm, open hands.

You see, I have renounced fear,
And over optimism, and expectation.
I will move ahead from here,
With a numbness tempered by determination, guts, patience,
And denial.

I will be smiling and singing all along,
And taking by horns of what comes my way,
With an unrelenting, aggressive battle cry.

Let's see what You "have in store" for me
For the ball is in Your court,
The Buck stops with You,
As I march forward, with a strong spirit,
And with all guns blazing.

The Tree of Purity

In today's modern age,
Where technology, competition, and pace,
Stand as the edifice of day-to-day lives,
People dive into this river of modernity,
Leaving behind their sensibilities, and sensitivity.

It is as though this river,
Brisk and rapid as it seems,
Washes away all that makes us human,
Purges us of our emotions, our feelings,
And hardens us into numbness,
A numbness that feels of uninhibited practicality.

But just like how an island emerges in the ocean,
A lotus blooms in a pond,
An oasis thrives in a desert,
The 0.1% that incompletes the 99.9%,
There are a fortunate few,
The chosen ones,
Who have souls that stand out
Like the rocks that stand in rivers.

Strong and mighty,
They stand unafraid,
Striking head-on into the river,
And ebbing the river away.
These rocks are the anomaly,
The unusuality,
The strange phenomena,
That are filled with souls,
Soft as feathers,
And hearts,
Made of Gold.

In this torrent of the river,
Stands a tough rock,
Small and inconsequential,
Shining with a luminescence,
Which outshines the stars,
And the shiny sun.

That stone,
the small, puny one,
the good-natured, purely soulful one,
the one with the golden core,
Is the one I call my mum.

A pure heart, an ethereal soul,
My mother is a tree,
That towers high above all,
In this garden of life.
Bearing ripe and juicy fruits,
That are plump with benevolence,
She is the tree that bears
Leaves greened with kindness.

All come and partake,
Of this wonder of nature-sown by Him Himself,
And she willingly embraces them,
With a cool shade of her warm purity.

There are a few some,
Like hunters, who climb upon her,
And fill their trunk of malevolence,
With a whiff of her goodness,
The Jealous Ones, they do inflict wounds,
That scar this innocent tree forever.

But just as goodness triumphs over evil,
Dawn succeeds darkness,

New leaves replace the dead ones,
And a flower blooms from a bud,
There she goes, standing tall,
With all grandiose and grandeur,
Shining ever-so-brightly,
My mother, in all her purity.

Me? I am just a branch on this tree,
Growing longer and thicker,
With leaves that are fragrant with
Insouciance.
This insouciance, is the water;
That the tree searches from the dark beneath,
And nourishes me with, lovingly.

There are storms when,
I shake vigorously and violently,
Trembling with fear and uncertainty,
When my mother has held on to me,
With the strong foundation,
Of motherly bond, love and bravery.

She has let many of her branches break,
To let me grow uninterrupted, undisturbed,
With a base that is,
As strong and resilient as her.

Mother, I promise you,
As I grow longer and stronger,
I will rise above and bend into the ground,
To support you even stronger.
When the storm comes,
Or when harm sways our way,
I will be the canopy,
That shades you from this grey.

We will withstand all together,
We will enjoy the spring,
We will bear our wondrous fruits,
And be the wonder we are.

Mother, you continue being evergreen as you are,
With your fragrance of sensitivity,
As you are one of the few trees,
That grow in this concrete garden of humanity.

I will stand by you,
Growing from you, into you,
And we will keep giving and partaking,
Our golden fruits of purity,
Our luscious fruits of humanity.

Halfway Down the Path Not Untaken

I was a very young boy then,
With not a care in the world,
Going through the prime of childhood,
Like any other would.

Standing at the end of the road,
Adolescence, as it is called,
I was about to change my track,
To the larger one called youth.

The road looked bright and attractive,
Like sunrise on the sea.
An aura you could not compare,
To any other reality.

Unfathomable are the ways of God,
He is a whimsical artist,
Who sways His brush as He wishes.

I was about to plant my feet,
On the lush, green track,
But I guess He had other plans for me,
For He chose to change my track.

This was like a typhoon,
Something that carries you away,
While you try to scamper about,
Trying to fight its might.

On a new path I fell upon,
A stark contradiction,
An anomalous antagonist,
To the path I was,
To step upon.

The path was very dark,
I would not say pitch black,
But it presented obstacles that were,
Mysterious and unknown at heart.

I tried to squint and survey,
The plan of this,
But failed to do so successfully,
You see, Time was not on my side.

And so, I began walking on this path,
With shaky fortitude,

That has been strengthened over time,
By determination, hope and
The implicit support of family.
This triumvirate is for me,
What a stick is to a limp,
What a guide is to the lost,
What brightness is to the dark,
And what a cradle is to a new-born.

Time and again this path has
Shaken and stirred me to the end,
It has presented adversities that are,
Herculean, to word in pen.

But just like a compass needle,
Which always points north
I have, time and again,
Struggled, withstood, fallen,
Picked myself up, and carried on.

Now, as I stand halfway down this path,
I have finally understood,
The nature of adversities,
As quoted by all.

You see, adversity is
A poison with its own antidote,
A thorn with its own red rose,
A mistake with its own moral lesson,
That always makes you realize,
Its profoundness at core.

God may be a whimsical artist,
Who sways His brush as He wishes,
But His canvas is always decorated,
With a painting full of purposefulness.

It is on this path that I have discovered,
Things that take years to fathom,
A self-rediscovery I would call it,
This path has given me a lot.

Time and Health are the most invaluable,
A value realized only by their absence,
The Human Spirit, tempered with Hope,

Is the strongest diamond formed,
These are some of the lessons,
This Ugly Guide has taught me.

Today as I stand on this path,
Trying to look ahead,
I don't know what lies in front of me,
So I look within.

Hope, Determination and Courage,
Are the sturdy boots
That will steer me forward,
On this long and bemusing path.

Rebirth

Wearing sturdy boots,
Of hope, determination and courage,
I was treading the path not untaken,
Hoping for its end, somewhere soon.

The road continued getting tougher,
Like ice freezing from water,
It had become a labyrinth of despair,
That continued to stretch forever.

It was then that I realized,
The viciousness that had caught me,
The inferno had begun to burn and melt,
The iron walls of my whole.

The sun of hope was on the horizon,
The sky of support had begun to dim,
My boots of resilience were wearing out,
And clouds of despair loomed within.

Frightened, and running out of fortitude,
I could only helplessly walk on,
Hoping hopelessly,
That this, too would pass along.

Maybe it was my destiny,
Maybe it was my karma,
Maybe it was The Whimsical Artist,
Who had swayed,
His brush again.

Another gush of typhoon,
Came and enveloped me,
While I again tried to fight,
Its powerful inevitable imminence.

This imminence threw me hard,
Roughly I landed on another path,
That caught me in its cradle,
And caressed the skirmishes,
That had almost broken me apart.

I squinted to survey,
The beauty of this newfound path,
A stark contradiction, an anomalous antagonist,
To the path I had fallen from.

'Purgatorio' as Dante called it,
The path was an ethereal bridge,
Steep and majestic in all its might,
Intimidating, but comforting,
This was the path to redemption,
To the Paradiso,
Of my lost friend,
Good health.

With hope as fresh as the morning dew,
Determination as fragrant as the wet earth,
Courage as strong as diamond,
I tightened my laces of patience,
And pulled up my socks of resilience,
To tread this path of certainty,
And re-unite with my mate.

A lot of inhabitants,
Who dwelled on the sidewalks,
Were my reliable guides,
Guiding me all the way.

Clad in milky white,
His angels would hold me
Every time I stumbled,
And cheer me every time I ran.

The path was not as smooth as silk,
It was a rough one,
But they were there to guide me,
And shelter me when I tired.

"Adversity is a poison with its own antidote."
"His canvas is always decorated with a painting full of
purposefulness."

Were the singers humming in my ears,
As I continued treading,
Towards a certain future
Guaranteed, as it was.

A rebirth I would call it,
Purgation of all
The Ugly Guide had offered,
A new whole had taken birth in me,
That would become my panacea.

Maybe God had seen enough,
Of the rigorous penance,
That fate had gifted me with,
And decided towards gifting a rebirth,
Of this new whole in me,
Thus, naming me Divyansh Atman.

Now, as I stand at the precipice of this path,
I truly understand,
The true nature of transience, as it always is.

What goes down always comes up,
The sun always rises after setting,
What breaks is always rebuilt,
Sufferings are like weak relations,
That are broken by the Iron Hand of Time.
These are some of the lessons,
This Angelic Cradle taught me.

With an additional layer of perspective,
My boots shine with new energy,
As I continue my sojourn,
Towards eternal heartiness and peace,
On this path, long, but not bemused.

She

Like a seed rupturing onto the surface,
Emerging into the sun,
Takes birth the ebullient cry,
Of the neonatal girl.

Jubilation and rejoicing
Are the pollen, spreading far and wide,
Shining in the motes of the sun,

Enlivening all,
With inherent invigoration.

"The Almighty has blessed us with a girl!"
"The female form has descended into our humble abode!"
Are the bellowing hallelujahs,
Reverberating out into the world,
Resounding with an undiminished resonance.

Eyes lively with curiosity,
Expressions painted with the explorer's chrome,
Limbs swinging like leaves in the wind,
Slowly she learns, and embraces,
The mortal world, hers to inhabit,
For the lifetime ahead.

Mother's flowering princess, Father's dear queen,
The apple of everyone's eye,
Delicately, quietly, innocuous,
Like the first petals of a flower,
She blooms—crawling and tumbling,
Drooling and shrieking,
Mumbling, rumbling and speaking,
Laughing, crying, to eventually walking,
Melting hearts with her childlike cuteness,
Enthralling everyone with her liveliness.

A voice, blessed twice with honey and sugar,
Gestures innate with the feminine,
She continues to grow and grow,
From tiny tot, into a young dame.

Enamouring everyone with beauty and elegance,
She goes about her life; free spirited, full spirited,
Laughing coyly in happiness,
Crying bitterly in sadness.

Inch-by-inch she plants her roots,
Into the soil of life,
Absorbing the vital nutrients of wisdom,
Negotiating, understanding the whimsical labyrinth,
Of worldly thoughts, worldly ways,

The virginal, pure dame,
Transforms into a refined lady,
Winning hearts with her womanish, slender disposition,
And defeating, quite a few,
As a femme fatale.

She is the golden fleece,
Suitors from far gather to woo,
Risking life, cheating death, wrestling the world,
Until the worthy she chooses.

A match made in heaven,
Tied by divine wishes,
An epoch cradles her consciousness,
Into a new, promising wonderland.

A new phase, a new chapter commences,
Frolicking and rollicking the couple progress,
Into lifetime companionship,
The Garden of Marriage.

Sweet love, mellow affection,
Mutual respect and understanding,
Tacit consensus, give-and-take,
Acquiescence, acknowledgement, utmost care,
Sacrifice, and dynamism,
Are the pearls encased,
In this oyster of wedlock-
Gently entering her soul,
As a wife's incarnate.

Old Father Time works His way,
Tacking and tocking through the day,
As she becomes a fruiting forest,
The breeder of the next gen.

A mother is born in the cradle of the child,
Bawling incessantly in her cuddling arms,
As she nurses and feeds the divinity,
Delivered by the divine into her embrace.

A cardinal emotion cultivates,
Into her heart, the cores of her being,
Unconditional love, motherly instincts,
Embroider themselves, into her conscience.

Raw and metaphysical grows the maternal gut,
Numbing, diluting other faculties,
Her life becomes a magnifying glass,
Omni focused on her child's most mundane moments.

A stream of irrational fears, insecurities and idiosyncrasies,
Irrigates this well,
As she becomes the hard shell,
Gently protecting, carefully nurturing,
The child, the essence her life.

The minutest of scratches, the tiniest of teardrops,
And there rages in her consciousness restlessly,
A blazing inferno she morphs into,
Comforting, consoling her child in the warmth,
While incinerating the cause to ashes.

Years and years pass,
Her child has now grown,
With his mother's parentage inscribes,
Into the deepest realms of his soul,

As the child sires his own,
Polishing her tresses into silvery notes.

Grandma she has become,
An alluring, warm, honeycomb.
Buzzing grandchildren flock,
To partake of her unending love,
A feathery kiss, a velvety pat,
Delightful surprises, Pandoraland of stories,
Are the sweet drops of honey,
The buzzers keenly thrive on.

She has seen a lot,
In this drama called life,
Cared for, loved deeply,
By the generation she is the seed of.
Sitting in her cradling chair,
Sighs impregnated with fulfilment,
Vision reflecting contentment,
She looks into her husband's eyes.

A mystical communication devoid of words ensues,
As they clutch their throbbing hands,
Ready to face,
The transient whim of change,
Accepting with full hearts
The inevitable nature of imminence.

The Mask

Behind those smug countenances,
And smiles over stretching the jaw,
Behind the sang froid reassurances,
And the expression of calm;
Behind the tough and resilient demeanour,

And the nonchalant, casual nature,
We lie, the people who use these as a mask,
Shrouding a pulsating universe.

The mask is illusionary, but convincing,
Convoluted and crafted into several avatars,
It is the hottest thing in vogue now-a-days,
Worn by one, and all.

Some wear it to hide,
The darkness and maliciousness trapped inside,
Feeding this ever-growing inferno,
Through genuine, 'gleaming' smiles,
Visible to the world,
As an amiable, warm shine.
Shining extremely bright on the surface,
Casting shadows of pitch black jealousy within,
On sensing happiness and good fortune of others,
Yearning wickedly, with extreme ominous desire,
For its conversion,
Into eternal misfortune.
A black hole is what resides in their heart,
Slowly consuming all existing goodness,
Every breath gasps of unsettling torment,
Slowly destroying them, and deeply hurting others.

Never can these people have peace of mind,
Haunted by a life with two faces.
Tear this mask, incinerate it,
Before it does the same to you.

Then there are others,
Using this mask as a tough, rugged shield
showing and convincing the world,
Of their strength, their contentment,

While defending, and protecting,
The throbbing vulnerability within.

Now there are two kinds in these,
Like two identical but distinctly different twins.
Both use this mask to protect themselves,
But one, to create a fictional avatar-
Full of personal aspirations and dreams;
While the other uses it,
As a cloud of denial—
Wanting oblivion,
From the internal, teeming adversity.

The former are merely living in an insidious bubble,
Magically woven by the very mask they created,
An impending doom, a hard shock awaits their conscious,
Accompanying the imminent burst.

The latter, protecting themselves,
Have a tough job on their hands,
For they need Herculean strength,
Withholding their only defence,
One chink, one give away, one lacuna
In the tough armour of their mask;
And there pierces the sword of worldly glares,
Brandishing pity, sharpened by despair,
Shooting fits of profuse pain,
Stripping the hidden abyss bare.

Don't let this mask be your master,
Make it your apprentice,
Use it as a shining diamond, if you have to,
Emanating your true persona, far and wide,
And not as a genie lamp,
To trap the true you,
That ought be out.

But why wear a mask,
Concealing the human soul within?
Let the true self radiate,
Unapologetically, unbarred, honest,
Into the wide, wide world.

There will always be the jury,
Of self-righteous hypocrites,
Whose whispers will linger on and on,
Like the subtle perfume of flowers-
That is not your worry.
For you are guided by YOUR conscience,
Not entangled in the draw strings,
The world wants it in.

And you listen only to YOUR inner voice,
Deaf to the misguiding whispers of the world.
You speak YOUR mind,
Untwisted and unfiltered,
By changing opinions, and varied expectations.

So go out, unmask yourself,
And show the world,
The fearless YOU! the real YOU!

Ayya

'Rosie' I had decided to call her,
A young child I was then,
As I was on the way to see her,
Innocently fearing lest she were dark.

Eyes as clear as water,
Gaze filled with motes of curiosity,
Cheeks as red as an apple,

Yes, she had a visage,
Personifying my name for her;
And an expression,
As innocent and tranquil as birth.

Quietly she learned how to crawl,
Like a flower blooming from a pod,
And cooing and gooing she learnt to pronounce,
Mummy, Papa and all,
There was only that one innocent word she uttered with a fault,
'Ayya', for bhaiya, of all.

We both grew up together,
Although half a dozen winters apart;
Laughing and playing, crying and fighting,
Learning and teaching, sleeping and waking,
As she twisted her tongue,
To move from 'Ayya' to 'Bhaiya'.
Today, she is a busy girl,
Hustling and bustling her way through the clock,
Humming and sauntering along,
And living life, as it was meant to be lived.
She might seem to one,
As a carefree, cool dunce,
A shy, inhibited one,
A not-so-smart, so-so girl;

But what does the world know,
Of the deep garden of profoundness,
Of the corals of wisdom,
Of the ocean of emotions,
She has within her?

'Incomparable delicate girl'- there is a reason why,
She has been christened thus,

Delicate and pure as a feather,
Incomparable and pristine as the coded threads,
That have shaped her as she is.

A soul designed to be pure,
A soul incapable of hurt,
A soul, delicate as the womb,
In which God gifted her to us.

Her expression is an enigma,
An enigma we can only partially understand,
Her words appear as normal as they are subtle;
A subtlety,
Understood only by us, an esoteric few.

Such innocence she possesses,
An innocence easily overcome,
By the tiniest of darkness,
Possessed by this wide, wide world.

I do believe,
Her feelings are a Pandora box,
That has gems and stones,
Locked and hidden from all of us.

Sometimes she does open it for me,
And mostly only to me,
Because I know the code to this box;
The word with which she first,
Called me.

It does sound strange,
A relation she could not word well initially,
Is the relation that is,
The one true pathway to her heart.

Oh my precious, lovely sister,
This elder sibling vows today,
In true sense and spirit,
To be the brother that
Deserves sisterly love as yours.

There is a reason why you let me explore,
The enigma of your core,
I do believe it is to be,
The protector, and guide,
Of the castle of your consciousness and conscience,
The thrones of which you are the queen.

I shall be the honourable knight that protects you,
The honourable teacher who guides you,
I shall be the kin that proves,
The identical nature of our blood.

Ayya, or Bhaiya,
This pen is proud and fortunate,
To have a sister as wonderful and special,
As is the divinity that has,
Made me a sibling of yours.

"Catch–Catch"

A brother and his younger sister,
Run along, hopping towards the garden,
To play 'catch–catch'.

No sooner did they reach,
a breeze began to blow,
Scented with earthy moistness,
Empowered by thundery belligerence.

Oblivious and carefree,
Unaware of the speeding gust,
They hopped along, hand in hand,
Heads bobbing, nodding.

The game of catch started,
She threw first, the ball cut the sharp wind,
With all strength that a child can muster;
Bouncing, swaying,
Striking at his boots.

"Yay!", "Well done!",
Both exclaimed,
While the trees gently swayed,
To the verdant, fresh innocence.

Perhaps Wily Wind wasn't pleased,
Speeding up, breathing deeper, hushing louder,
A storm gathered until when,
Dark, daunting, despairing.
The siblings did get scared,
The strands of their hair, trembling in the gushing air,
Crying louder than the laughing thunder.

But 'catch–catch' was a game not new to them,
Played comfortably, enjoyed in equal measure,
Immune to the vagaries,
Of wicked weather.

So the siblings go on and on,
Throwing the ball to each other,
Catching, and returning it with triumph,
While Wicked Weather and Wily Wind
Stand perplexed, watching the marvel,
That is sibling unity.

So here we go, sister,
I have held the ball a long time,
Admiring it, tossing it vertically,
While your eager, yet patient eyes look on,
Curious for the next throw.

I am throwing the ball to you,
Catch it.
Admire it, spin it, bounce it, head it,
Until you've had your fill
Of fun,
Languidly trying to soothe the longing,
Distance and time that separates us from.

Hold on to the ball for me,
While I tie my shoe laces,
Adjust my cap, knocked off by the wind,
And steady my stance,
Shaken by fickle fate.

Dearly Departed

Dear departed,
Look at what is left,
Named as your remnants.

The soul has left its home,
Sudden as your departure.
Marks of your legacy overwritten,
By selfish kin itself.

Strange is the depth of your mark,
Fluttering far and wide,
Unable to hold the fort,
At its very home.

Those blessed of the doting,
Showered relentlessly by you,
Have forgotten it seems,
Memories, of your remembrance.

Fault lies in them,
Shrouding in oblivion,
What you left behind.
Guilty are they of contempt,
Defacing innocence and greatness,
Commanded by you.
Dear departed,
We were kept apart,
By time and tide,
Your love, your memory,
Breaks the dubious labyrinth,
Spun by fate.

You will forever thrive,
In conscience, in actions, in visage.
Respect and honour you will enjoy,
Thriving in the realm,
Bowed in your memory.

The Powerful and the Powered

Shaky stance,
Trembling silhouette,
The powered stands,
Patiently, insignificantly.

Stretching every sinew,
Craning, squinting,
The powered looks on,
Hopefully, hopelessly,

For an approving nod, for a genial acceptance,
Treading pillar to post,
Mind bent on accomplishment.

Violent pushes, tumbling pulls,
Raucous pandemonium,
Pass through its constitution,
As it barely places its hands,
On the majestic cliff—
Where power resides.

An imposing countenance,
Embodiment of aura,
Asserting dominance and strength,
There sits power, with nonchalance,
On the throne decorated, built from the bricks,
Of which aspirations and expectations are flecks.
An imposing visage,
Brazed with smug shades,
Power looks on aggressively,
Over his proud nose,
Gleaming with status, exhibiting his ego.

"What want you?" Dances in the void,
Choreographed by swagger, supercilious in tempo,
The beats slowly rain down,
Reaching the powered,
Ears are the barren land of.

Humble, hesitant prayers,
Flap out, with weak strides,
Dusting, brushing the robe.

Shaking, reverberating with prayer,
They tingle the sole,
Power lay his foot upon.

"It isn't my bother",
"Go have cake if you can't have bread"
Are the cuts piercing gingerly,
Into the sturdy wall,
The powered cements resolve on.
A seed has just been sown,
A spark has just been kindled,
Growing, raging,
Feeding on the arrogance,
The power is so stubborn of.

A wildfire, it turns to ash,
The very foundation of the throne,
Tumbling to the cursing ground,
With an ignominious groan.

A tower made of wooden sticks,
Comes cascading down,
With the same pace,
At which it was built.
Watched woefully by the elder brother
Whose name is Responsibility.

A long mane, grey with wisdom,
A stance speaking of righteousness,
Eyes filled with an ethos,
He nods his head in dismay.

"Such a shame."
Are the sullen words,
Exhaled in the sigh,
He breathed out.
Power and Responsibility,
Are inseparable brothers,
The powered rest upon whom,
Delicate dreams, and trembling arms.

Corruption, the insidious mistress,
Waves her irresistible charm,
A honey trap awaits Power,
Dare he take a mouthful from.

"Nooooo!" wails the prudent one,
Despair strikes whom,
As he watches his beloved brother,
Entranced, and consumed,
Into absolution.

The Introvert

A face as blank as a sheet,
A voice as feeble as a kitten's,
There treads the Introvert,
Shrugging shoulders, and drooping all along.

Eyes as nervous as a lamb's in a slaughterhouse,
Gestures as tentative as the weather,
The Introvert is like a cat,
Moving as stealthily as silence,
Breathing as weakly as before a yawn.

Admiration and yearning are all their eyes speak,
Seeing charisma, warmth and amiability.
"Oh! How I wish that I was!"
silently, the Introvert screams on.

Like the greens in a desert,
Are the few friends of this creature,
Who feels like a fish out of the water,
When pushed into the tropical rainforest,
Of hustle, bustle, laughs, claps, slaps,
And all that the Introvert is not.

The Introvert, to an Extrovert,
Is a stiff, ungenial snob,
The pillow to prick the thorn,
The specimen to try pranks on.
But, don't ever be mistaken,
What shows, is not what is,
The Introvert is a world in itself,
A world, unique and profound.
A plethora of Intelligence,
A river of thoughts,
A sea of emotions,
And an ocean of fun,
Is what the Introvert hides,
Under the brown, fibrous fort.

An Introvert is its own best friend,
Its own sound judge,
Who can analyse, a persona,
With just a whiff of talk.

One line uttered by an Introvert,
Has five internal aliters,
Uttering the best of the lot,
The most euphemistic of them all.

A dynamic thinker is an Introvert,
Whose mind is like a lightning bolt,
Ever-running, ever-thinking,
Never resting, and never idling.
Fun is alone-time for it,
Dancing alone, humming alone,
Such an introvert, an Introvert is,
That its mind is a never ending boom-box,
Playing symphonies from memory,
Never missing a song.

It possesses eidetic memory,
Remembering the minutest of motes,
Of all that it sees, hears, speaks,
And experiences every day.

You might be thinking,
"What nonsense is this?"
"Gibberish rantings!"
"Random stuff!", et al.
But, mind you, my friends,
This pen is one,
A proud Introvert, asserting it,
Overwhelmingly, on the inside,
And timidly, on the outside.

Introverts, be proud (be shy),
You are a shining mote (a dim shadow),
Unapologetic, uninhibited (apologetic, inhibited),
And an Extrovert (an Introvert),
Within (on the outside).
That's all.

Priority's Play

A curious case of truant,
Always subject to whim,
Haughtily saunters priority,
Chuffing, scoffing away.

Blissful are the ways it sways,
Trampling, stifling the loom of fate.
An absence of regard, a deficiency of rationale,
Maul the visages,
Sway upon whom it may.

Groaning, gasping in disarray,
One and all witness in helplessness,
While priority sets upon its play,
Dismantling, disjoining, rejoining,
The mangled clay,
Life that trades as.

An inquisitive child it is,
Let it play.
Beat and shape it the toddler will,
Into a masterpiece,
Of sense, and rationale.

The loom of fate will be the enrapturing embroidery,
Enshrining this eccentricity,
Budding and mature becomes when the genius,
Notorious as priority's play.

Blood Is Thicker than Water

Blood is thicker than water.
But some are thinners like aspirin.
While vital electrolytes are few in those,
Not sharing the same blood.

The aspirin provides relief no doubt,
Soothing, calming, relieving.
Consume too much,
And things could fall apart.

The electrolytes are vital elixir,
Time and again infused they,
Fortify, strengthen, rejuvenate,
Conscience, consciousness and spirit.

Aspirin, restrained by need,
Electrolytes, parched runs whenever,
The mental compass is disillusioned, giddy,
Will set charter in good stead,
The essential twins-
State of mind,
Peace of soul.

The Grass Is Greener on the Other Side

The grass is greener on the other side,
That which is not ours,
Shines bright,
Captivating, bedazzling,
The innocent, oblivious eye.

"Oh! How I wish that I had!",
Exclaims the desirous foolish mind,
Disregarding dear possessions,
Shrouded in the shadow,
Of the shine and verdancy,
Replete on the other side.

The mind is an infant,
Jumping and drooling about,
Smoke and mirrors;
Relinquishing the cardinal lesson,
Not everything that glitters is gold.

Oh innocent mind!
What thou hast,
Is the glitter for the other,
Desirous of whose possessions,
Thou art.

A cunning crook desire is,
Wielding razzle-dazzle,
Enticing the mind,
Into a labyrinth of nothingness.

Bat away this desire with contentment,
Respect and love are the moist drops,
Greenery that paint,
Onto all our possessions;
Bringing a gleam greener,
Than on the other side.

Diwali

With the might of a lightning bolt,
Struck the arrow of good,
Into the heart of the evil,
The evil, the mighty, intimidating evil,
Falling, and dissolving,
With the same power,
As it hath possessed.

An epoch it was,
A new message had been born,
And cradled across all the realms and directions,
"Goodness has triumphed over evil", loud and clear,
Seeped into the conscious of every being.

Those who despaired, those who trembled,
With an uncertain fear,
Hath now known,
This lore of victory,
Of righteousness, over tyranny.

Radiant smiles radiated everywhere,
Spreading like wildfire,
People rejoiced and sang,
With a newfound conscience,
That would guide them,
Towards the path of good karma, and moksha.
Candles were lit, houses blushed with jubilance,
The sky had a rich hue and glow,
Of all that was, and is, good,
Warding off the darkness,
Of all that was, and is, bad.

The festival of lights comes and goes,
Year after year after year.
Candles dance in the wind,
Diyaas glitter with golden prosperity,
The earth smiles colourfully,
And sweets of joy and festivity,
Flow like the river, during rain.

Year after year after year,
This is how Diwali comes and goes,
Coming in with sweets and presents,
Going out with fireworks and prayers.
But there is one thing,
This Diwali brings us every year,
And that thing is not just any other thing,
But a value, most valuable,
Whose value is invaluable.

Today in the Kal-Yug (The Dark Age),
This day is a testament,
That the dark can never conquer the light,
The light of knowledge, the light of righteousness, the light of
principles,

Which is the triumvirate,
That will burn bright, and radiant,
For eternity, and through eternal darkness.

This Diwali, unleash this trinity within you,
And let it burn with omnipotence.
Kindness is the light that will spread,
Goodness is the crackle that will echo,
Happiness is the warmth that will spread,
Inviting all the comfort of contentment,
Enriching all the conscience possessed,
And being fuelled by blessings, from those,
The flame hath touched.

Blaze

Two stones struck together,
By a chance as minute,
As a candle's in a storm,,
There arose a bright amber spark,
Engulfing all the darkness there was.

With fear and awe witnessed this wonder,
Man, animal, and all,
As it turned brighter and lighter,
Stronger and warmer,
Inviting, and warning all.

A courage shaking with fear,
He approached it, uncertain, but sure,
this new wonder of nature,
Had been born as his new companion.

Slowly he wielded and learnt,
The fire, burning bright and hot,

Using it, as it was meant,
Adding new strength to all known so far.

There came a point in time,
When he made the blazing breath so hot,
That it swallowed him,
And those,
Who enraged it so much.

Some worship it,
Some stay away from it,
Everyone needs its warmth,
An accidental serendipity it may be,
But it is not that, at all.

The fire that glows so bright and radiant,
Resides inside all of us.
Burning bright when called for,
Burning dim when not.

It is this fire,
That invokes passion, courage and determination;
And it is also this same fire,
That invokes pride, anger, jealousy, and hatred,
When fuelled by the darkness,
That lurks around our human soul.

Nerves of steel,
A rock-strong resilience,
Burning determination,
Radiant visage,
Are all the various traits,
Carefully tested by this Master,
Who can burn those who give up,
And strengthen those who don't.

Look into the fire, my friends,
Look at its profoundness,
And rekindle the fire in you,
To make the spirit strong,
Stronger than ever before.

The Ecstasy of Expectation

I was lost, deep,
In the waves of subconsciousness,
Swimming through the lagoons of slumber.

The body was resting, recharging, and
Getting ready for a new day.
And then, it happened.
I had an epiphany.

How quaint that feeling was,
A moment hard to describe,
The thought was like a burst of flavour,
On an otherwise bland pie.

It was like a pattern,
On an otherwise blank slate,
That shimmers and then disappears,
Just to draw your head.

You must be wondering,
What is this sentimental fool,
Going on, writing and scribbling?
Patience is a virtue,
A virtue I most respect,
I will reveal what I am ranting about.
At once, right away.
I was in the stage of slumber,

When the mind is in the deepest realm of sleep,
When the mind usually conjures,
Dreams that are too strong to leave.

Ironically, my mind was completely blank,
Something that I did not quite realize,
Only to have this flash of epiphany.
An epiphany
Of a happy reunion.

The Deviant One just veered off,
Like a piece of paper in the wind,
To a land where I found myself,
Among faces very familiar to me....

....It were those same visages,
I had spent many a happy moment with,
Their company is a canoe,
Sailing in the waves of tranquillity.

Laughing, joking, teasing and smiling,
We exchanged our pleasantries,
The canoe bobbed with the vibration,
Of the reunion, so comforting.

The feeling, which was too short,
To be actually termed a dream,
Was like a drop of water,
In an otherwise dry stream.

It was that sprinkle of dew, the sprinkle of moistness,
Which rouses you out of sleep,
Only to make you fresh and ask,
My, what was it??

Oh my dear,
How much I have missed your company,
How much I have craved reminiscence,
How strong these feelings are,
They just daunt me,
When I had this beautiful epiphany.
I would like to call it,
The ecstasy of expectation.
A beautiful feeling, that cute little expectation.
It is like a comfortable, cosy cushion,
For the very tired mind,
To rest on, once in a while,
And unwind momentarily.

This morning I realized,
The beauty and power of this feeling.
a feeling that helps the mind,
Cling to the most pure and beautiful,
Of memories.

I don't know when the reunion will occur again,
Although I know about its inevitability,
But, Oh, expectation,
Thanks a ton!
For taking me to the perigee,
Of this reality,
Like a magician toying with illusion.

It is really hard to describe,
Was that....illusion or reality?
But, I can most certainly assert,
Expectation, you enthralled me.

The "Cupple"

Accompanying Old Mrs Sunshine,
As ravishing and fresh as in her youth,
They descend—
Boiling, brewing and blending,
Into the abode of people;
With refreshing, effervescent countenances,
And enticing, invigorating warmth.

Meet the "Cupple"
Arriving with swagger—
The charming, dynamic, flamboyant
Mr Cocoa Robusta,
And clutching his arm,
Sauntering in the most dainty of ways,
The demure, the bedazzling,
Mrs Flora Foliage.

Mr Robusta—
With a masculine cologne,
Rousing to full attention,
The stubbornness of slumber,
Takes a dive into the steaming sauna,
Bubbling impatiently for a strong embrace,
Into his alluring ruggedness.

A tantalising aroma,
A refreshing effervescence,
Materialises from the kettle.
Like a ghost it lurks and wanders,
Wearing a perfume,
Humming, and whistling of cocoa beans,
Kindling the twigs of olfaction.

In another kettle close by,
Swimming with grace,
Good enough to make a mermaid look pale,
Mrs Flora Foliage, all subtle and delicate,
Enlivens the aqua,
With strokes of her mellow scent,
And dabs of her herbal shades.

A meadow, verdant, and ambrosial,
Grows into the waking consciousness,
Tingling the sluggish slumber,
Into animated sprightliness.

"Good morning!", "Have a nice day!",
Sing melodiously onto the cheerful visages,
Partaking from the ebullient "Cupple"
The cynosure of the conversation table.

The "Cupple"—
Are the heralds of the day,
Giving an encouraging push,
To conquer the new day,
Gently lullabying the yawning, and sprouting laze.

What would we be without them—
Slumbering and drooling through the day?
Let us raise a toast in grace,
To this couple, every day.

His Name Personifies Him

Like the first rays of the sun,
He gets up with conviction,
Ready to face the world, which presents,
New challenges, offers new opportunities-

With fresh courage, fresh hope,
And fresh determination.
His name personifies him.

Every day he boots himself up,
And heads into the awakening lap of Mother Nature,
The chirping of birds, the rustling of leaves,
The feel of countless motes, enlivened in the sun,
The symphony of sea waves,
Are his morning friends,
Who give him the momentum,
To face the daunting day.
His name personifies him.

After seeing off his daughter to school,
He returns home to a warm cup of tea,
Served with bellows of laughter, talks and discussion,
Made exclusively with affection and care,
by his spouse.
And that's all he takes,
Before going to dress himself up,
To face his boss, the day.
His name personifies him.

With lunchbox in hand, and calmness in mind,
He reaches his office, always on time.
He sits there on his chair, working with full dedication,
Always being respected by his subordinates,
And admired by his higher ups, and coordinates,
Talking to everyone with all courtesy and respect,
He is strict, but not rigid,
Firm, but not rough,
Respectful, but not sycophantic,
Understanding, but not gullible,
Organized, but not fascist,

And, above all, dignified, but not foolish.
With all these tools in hand, he carries on his work
And aims to fulfil it, at that place, at that time.
His name personifies him.

He rings the doorbell, only to see his lively family,
And savours his morning "diet" again,
He goes to teach his daughter and oversee his boy's studies,
And, after accomplishing it, yawns with a mouthful of
contentment and relief,
Only to fall fast, fast asleep.

This might sound very "ordinary",
To a person who is not aware,
Of the trials and tribulations,
In his daily life.
What if I were to tell you, my friends,
Of his responsibilities,
Steep as the mountains they are?
Of the predicaments and misfortunes,
That have struck him all at once, like thunder and lightning?
Of the most mundane to the most monumental of tasks,
like hydrogen atoms and stars, he fulfils regularly?
What if I were to tell you all this, indeed,
And tell you, also,
That he does all this,
Coolly, calmly, with all sang froid,
Smilingly, happily, without a sign of complaint,
Sincerely, whole-heartedly, without slackness,
Uncompromisingly, with balance, without collateral damage,
And yet finds plenty of time,
for himself and his family??
What if?

Time is the strongest and the most perpetual witness,
Of ALL this man does,
He is a master of resourcefulness, a true task-manager,
Who works as efficiently as a racing car,
But bettering it,
With his ethereal touch of humanity.
His name personifies him.
Now, doesn't he look colossal?
Living, as he is, with all guile, guts and gristle?
But the beauty lies in the fact, as all good things go,
In his simplicity, his dignity.
"If you can walk with kings, nor lose the common touch"
Oh Kipling! How true art thou whilst saying this.....
His name personifies this.

As someone who lives,
Under the aegis of his shadows,
Always protected, always carefree,
Idolizing him, deifying him,
I, my friends, have lots to say about him,
Yet, I am speechless.

What not can one learn from him...
He is an institution in himself, a true inspiration,
The choicest of virtues, the most golden of personalities
Are gilded in him.
He is, like an umbrella,
Who protects all those under him,
In the rain of challenges,
He is that shining star,
Who assumes a rather modest pedestal,
But is helpless,
Because his personality shines in him, and illuminates,
His vicinity.
His name personifies him.

Oh, Master-craftsman,
I did not know,
You were so dextrous, so skilled,
That your craft is so good.
He is, to you, and to us,
What Mona Lisa is to Da Vinci,
What David is to Michelangelo,
What the Apostles are to Jesus,
What Bhagwad Gita is to the righteous,
What music is to the musician,
And what life is to the living.
His name, is, truly, a true personification of him.

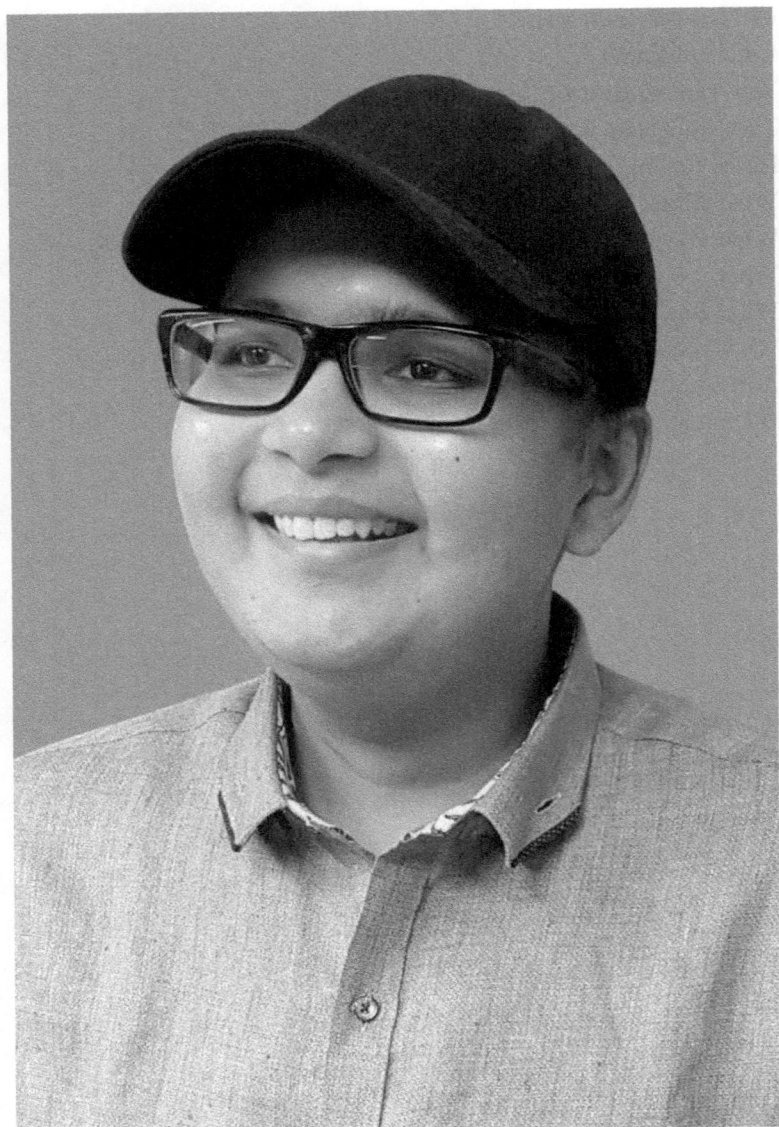
Divyansh Atman